ROAD MAP TO HEALTH

7 Steps to Alter Your Destination

STACEY J. ROBINSON, MD

Krista!
Wishing you abundant!
health & wellness!
Stacey
1-3-19

Henry & Aubrey Publishing LLC
200 Central Avenue, Suite 810
Saint Petersburg, FL 33701

www.RobinsonMed.com

Editors: Casey Cavanagh, Ke'Shawnda Chambers, Monica San Nicolas, Patti Porzig, Judy Hotchkin, and Diane Graham

Cover design by Valerie Bogle

First Edition: September 2015

ISBN: 0998400807

ISBN-13: 978-0998400808

This book is dedicated to my family.

To my parents: Thank you for raising me to believe in my dreams.

To my children, Davis & Casper: You are my world.

_____

To the world you may be one person;

But to one person you may be the world.

~ Author Unknown

ACKNOWLEDGMENTS

I would like to express my deepest gratitude to the following people, who made this book possible.

My Family & Friends—My beautiful children, Davis and Casper. Thank you for putting up with all the time that I spent researching, writing and editing this book. And to my mom, my sister, Diane, and my good friend Patti for reviewing and editing the book. And to all my friends for giving me feedback on the title and cover.

My Patients—You inspired me to write this book by trusting me with your health, sharing your struggles, and most importantly, asking challenging questions that inspire me to learn more and more each day.

The Incredible Staff at Robinson MD—Sheila Floyd, Sierra Watson, Karen "K.C." Cox and Kristen Jones. Your dedication to providing excellence in medicine goes above and beyond expectations. Special thanks to Jo Brower for having the faith to join me at the beginning of the journey and helping to lay the groundwork for our mission.

My Business Coaches—My coach, Barb Kyes, as well as Ford and Juliet Kyes at ActionCOACH Tampa Bay. Thank you for keeping me "above the line," showing me how to be a leader and business owner and keeping me focused on my "why." And a big thank you to all the Quantum Leap coaches who taught me how to tell my story and fine-tune my book.

My Graphic Designer—Valerie Bogle. Thank you for creating a beautiful cover and for having patience with me during the design process.

The Institute for Functional Medicine (IFM)—This trailblazing organization makes the practice of Functional Medicine possible for physicians to pave the way for a new and better way to practice medicine.

The Pioneers—All the physician authors listed in the Resources who showed me that it is possible to be an author and practice medicine.

CONTENTS

INTRODUCTION

Take care of your body. It's the only place you have to live.

~ Jim Rohn

If you are looking for better health and vitality, seeking ways to avoid chronic diseases, and want to understand what may be triggering your symptoms, you have come to the right place.

Back in 2007, I was working for a large HMO organization, seeing a patient every ten minutes in a busy outpatient clinic. I remember walking into the sterile exam room to see yet another new patient, my fourth of the morning. Already 45 minutes behind, I only had time to glance at her name and date of birth. She was just a few years my senior, but appeared much older. Her gray hair framed a round face and the baggy clothes attempted to hide the 15 pounds she had gained since her last visit.

She came in with a long list of medical problems and an even longer list of medications. Her medical "problem list" was simply a list of symptoms and syndromes—irritable bowel syndrome, depression, high blood pressure, high cholesterol, reactive airway disease, allergies, and more. Writing out prescription after prescription, I tried to glance up from my prescription pad while we got acquainted. I did a quick examination, reviewed blood work with her, and handed her the thick pile of prescriptions.

As I said good-bye, reached out my hand, and touched the doorknob, she said quietly, "Dr. Robinson, I forgot to tell you that I have been having some heartburn for the past few months." I looked at the clock and saw that I was almost an hour behind and still hadn't finished with half of my morning patients. I asked her a few quick questions and prescribed an acid blocker. I knew the medication would eliminate her symptoms; however, I also knew that the drug wouldn't address the underlying problem. I was mad at myself for just putting a Band-Aid on her symptoms, but I had no time to delve into a really in-depth health history to help her.

As I watched her walk down the hallway, I suddenly felt an overwhelming sense of frustration and sadness. I'm not sure why it happened at that moment. Maybe my frustration with the broken system in which I was trapped collided with seeing her walking out with yet another bottle of pills. Or maybe it was just my realization of the increasingly futile nature of the way in which I was now practicing medicine.

The sheer volume of patients I had to see each day did not allow for the time to truly help people get to the root cause of their problems. I felt exhausted, frustrated, sad, and hopeless for the future of medicine. This isn't what I envisioned when I was in medical school. I had a deep desire to help people transform their health, but I felt handcuffed by the medical establishment and was nearing burnout.

Not long after, I remembered an article I had read that got my attention at the time. That doctor described a model of care called direct-care practice, that was reminiscent of the days of Marcus Welby MD—the days before insurance and HMOs. I had set it aside with a faint thought that maybe I could try it someday. Well, that day had arrived—enough was enough. I decided I would take the plunge and break free from the medical system underlying our chronic disease epidemic.

After ten years of practicing medicine within the confines of the insurance-driven health-care system, I jumped ship and started a concierge/direct-care practice. I stopped accepting insurance and patients now pay me directly. This wasn't a decision that I took lightly—it took several years of contemplation and introspection. I had to deal with the guilt of abandoning my colleagues who were struggling through a dysfunctional system. Most importantly, I had to make sure it was the right decision.

Ultimately, I decided that the health-care system was unlikely to be fixed within my lifetime. I realized I could make a more significant contribution by caring for a few hundred patients exceptionally well rather than caring for thousands of patients poorly. I knew I would be of little use to anyone—my patients or my family—if I continued down a road toward burnout. I decided I could help patients truly heal if I could develop a practice which brought back the earlier days of a healthy, caring doctor-patient relationship.

In 2008, I opened a practice that began simply with me, my laptop, my cellphone, and my checkbook. I started from scratch with no patients, just a big dream of a better way to practice medicine. One at a time, people began showing up at my door. As I started treating them, it was not long before I rediscovered my love of medicine and how precious TIME can be in the world of healing. Not only did I rediscover my passion for medicine, I soon began pursuing alternative ways to help people to identify and treat the earliest signs of imbalance and to prevent disease through Functional Medicine, which deals with the root cause of chronic disease.

In this book you will learn about Functional Medicine, a new and rapidly growing medical approach revolutionizing the landscape of medicine. More and more doctors are embracing this approach, breaking free of the limitations of conventional medicine. And patients are discovering that there is a way to healing that lies outside the pharmaceutical industry. In 2014, the respected Cleveland Clinic opened a Center for Functional Medicine, a definitive sign that this innovative way of practicing medicine is spreading to the mainstream.

Stacey J. Robinson, MD

After 20 years as a practicing physician, I know our health is determined mostly by our lifestyle. We desperately need to return to the basic premises of health, such as nutritious food, increased movement, plenty of sunshine, sufficient sleep, and relaxation. My goal in writing this book is to provide you with a field guide to health, outlining a simple plan that is realistic and practical. Here you will also find essential resources at your fingertips that you can use today to make the best choices for your health.

In *Road Map to Health,* you will encounter powerful stories about how people took control and changed their health. You will read about remarkable medical studies which demonstrate how powerful changes in lifestyle can be as effective as medications in treating numerous diseases. You will discover how to become healthier by tweaking your daily choices. Finally, the guidance in this book will unleash the motivation that you need to change your habits and reach your best possible health.

So let's get started making simple, daily changes that will change your future health for the better.

PART I—A REVOLUTIONARY NEW APPROACH TO HEALTH

Stacey J. Robinson, MD

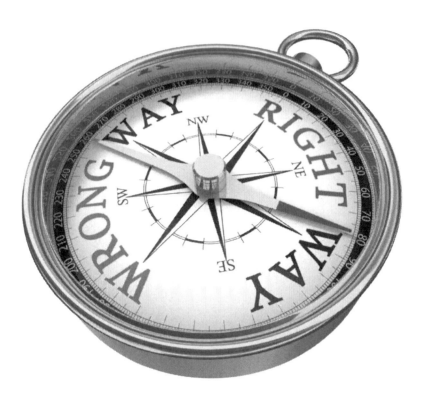

CHAPTER ONE

WHY WE ARE HEADED IN THE WRONG

DIRECTION

America has an epidemic of chronic disease. We are fortunate to have what is arguably the best, most technologically advanced health-care system in the world. Yet the incidence of chronic disease continues to rise in epidemic proportions—obesity, heart disease, diabetes, autoimmune disease, cancer, and dementia. Compared to 11 developed countries, the United States has dropped to dead last when it comes to overall health.[1]

In conventional medicine, the approach is to categorize patients with a disease and match the disease to a medication or surgical treatment, often just masking the symptoms rather than fixing the dysfunction. The right approach, outlined in this book, is to find the imbalances and fix disease at the root cause.

Many factors play into this chronic disease epidemic. One is the financial conflict of interest of industries that heavily influence medicine.

The Pharmaceutical Industry

Arguably the most powerful player in health care, "Big Pharma" has enormous political and social power, influencing every aspect of medicine. The pharmaceutical industry filled 4 billion prescriptions in 2014, equating to nearly $374 billion.[2] A "pill for every ill" exists and most Americans have bought into this quick-fix, prescription-writing approach to their health.

A whopping 70 percent of Americans take at least one daily medication. Even more shocking, 20 percent take five or more daily medications.[3] I don't want to minimize the importance of medications—some are lifesaving, especially those used for life-threatening conditions. For chronic disease, though, medications are not always the solution. Despite this dependence on medications, America has some of the highest rates of cancer, heart disease, dementia, diabetes, and obesity in the world.

The sad part is that while roughly 80 percent of chronic disease is preventable and treatable through lifestyle measures, our health-care system largely ignores these powerful preventive and treatment options.[4] The primary focus of conventional medicine is on the treatment of disease with medication and surgery. And probably deep down, we all know this is not the right approach. However, changing an enormously profitable system will not be easy. Prescribing medications for chronic disease without fixing the underlying cause creates lifelong pharmaceutical industry customers. In this book, you will learn the powerful ways that your lifestyle choices can help you to avoid becoming one of them.

The Food Industry

Although you wouldn't normally think of the food industry in connection with health care, "Big Food" has an enormous impact on Americans' health. There is no question that this industry giant contributes to our chronic disease epidemic. The food industry is a TRILLION dollar business. And like Big Pharma, Big Food is in the business of creating lifelong customers.

Food companies create food-like substances made up primarily of a proprietary blend of sugar, fat, salt, and other "natural flavors" that keep customers wanting more. For example, studies show sugar stimulates the same areas of the brain as addictive drugs, like cocaine, releasing endorphins and dopamine, which leads to a powerful physical addiction.[5]

In addition to their addictive properties, these processed foods are devoid of the important nutrients your body needs to function optimally and are also filled with harmful chemicals used to improve shelf life.

Processed convenience foods are creating generations of people who don't know how to cook or prepare foods from scratch. Many of our children don't know where real food comes from, since the majority of what we eat is highly processed and comes out of a box, bag, can, or frozen package. It's not really food, but deconstructed components of real food put back together in colorful, fun, convenient packages. It is really more of a food-like substance than real food—or, as Dr. Mark Hyman refers to them, "Frankenfoods."[6] And they are slowly poisoning us.

This book will give you scientific proof that food is medicine. I will walk you through principles to help you identify foods that heal and avoid foods that are harming you. And I will provide you with resources and simple ideas to help you choose foods that provide the fuel, energy, and building blocks your body needs to function optimally.

Medical Education

So just how are medical doctors educated to practice medicine? We are taught to be great diagnosticians. This is the "holy grail" of medical school—to be great at making a diagnosis—and the entire medical education revolves around this process. We are taught to look for a pattern of symptoms and label patients with a disease. We are so focused on naming the disease that we don't consider why the patient is sick in the first place.

Physicians are also taught "practice guidelines" to treat each disease; these published documents outline the most effective and proven treatments. The algorithms are published by various organizations and made available to physicians. In theory, this sounds like a good thing, but it promotes categorizing patients with a disease and treating all of those patients with the same treatment plan regardless of the cause. Practice guidelines are so pervasive that doctors can easily lose sight of the fact that one so-called "disease" can have many different root causes. And the majority of treatments listed in these recommendations are medications.

Conventional medicine is based on an organ-specific approach, rather than looking at the body as a whole with each organ system working together to create health. This creates a philosophy focused on patients like they're a box of parts. We have a specialist for each body part: a cardiologist to treat our heart, a neurologist to treat our brain, a gastroenterologist to treat our gut, an orthopedist to treat our joints, a pulmonologist to treat our lungs, etc. So who is looking at the big picture?

The doctor who should be viewing the system as a whole is our primary care physician: the internist, pediatrician, or family doctor. In theory, this also sounds good, but in practice, it doesn't work very well. First, most medical schools don't teach this whole-body approach. Like the specialists, a primary care physician also treats each organ as if it were a separate entity. Second, in our insurance-based model of reimbursement, primary care specialties don't have enough face-to-face patient time to provide this comprehensive type of care.

This book focuses on a new and better approach: Functional Medicine. It looks at the body as a whole, with organs working together to keep the entire system in balance. This philosophy focuses on identifying the root cause of disease—all the factors involved (genetics, environment, and lifestyle)—and working toward correcting the imbalance.

The Insurance Industry

The primary care physician is not valued as important. This is reflected in the low insurance reimbursement of primary care specialties, which doesn't allow your doctor the time needed to care for you as a whole patient. Low reimbursement for primary care physicians limits the time they have available to care for you and forces them to see a large volume of patients. The average primary care doctor cares for more than 2,300 patients.[7] This important "quarterback" of your health becomes only a "gatekeeper," passing off to each specialist because they don't have enough time to know and care for that many people.

Furthermore, the many specialists treating the patient rarely communicate with each other about how the diseases are connected, or how their prescribed treatment affects the rest of the body. They often don't communicate with the primary care physician who referred you to them, either. We look to our family doctors for advice, but they are so encumbered by the large volume of patients and by providing codes and documentation to the insurance company that they don't have time to practice medicine in an effective way.

Health insurance in America reimburses physicians and hospitals for treating and managing disease, not for promoting health. Reimbursement depends on a diagnosis code, encouraging the practice of labeling patients with a disease. Insurance pays for "encounters," not prevention. It pays for medications and surgeries, not nutrition and lifestyle counseling. Unfortunately, powerful treatments using food, exercise, and relaxation are largely ignored and almost never prescribed—because insurance doesn't reimburse for it.

Maybe we need to change our own perspective on insurance and start investing in our own health. Insurance should be used for catastrophic, unexpected expenses, not maintenance of our health. We wonder why health insurance is so expensive. How expensive would our automobile insurance be if we demanded it paid for oil changes and tire rotations and other services that keep our car "healthy"? Yet, that is what we expect from health insurance.

I will show you how you can invest in your health as a way to prevent chronic disease and empower you to keep yourself healthy. We all need health insurance to cover those unexpected illnesses; however, we shouldn't rely on the insurance industry to determine what is best for us from a prevention standpoint.

Jan's Story

When Jan first came to see me, she was 55 years old and had been struggling with multiple sclerosis (MS), an autoimmune disease affecting the brain and nervous system, since her late 20s. Her health had deteriorated to a point where she envisioned herself becoming physically disabled. Going up and down the stairs was becoming increasingly difficult and she was afraid she would have to sell the home she loved. She was desperate to find answers that she was not getting from conventional medicine.

Jan felt poorly all the time. She was seeing many specialists and taking nine prescription medications, including a powerful immune-suppressing drug for her MS. She already took two drugs to lower her blood pressure and was getting ready to start a third. Intolerable pain and muscle spasms required her to take a variety of prescriptions to ease her symptoms, including antidepressants, muscle relaxants, and medications for nerve pain. These drugs only masked the symptoms and had a variety of unpleasant side effects.

The daily heartburn, bloating, and constipation she had experienced most of her life were signs that her gut was not healthy, but the only answer conventional medicine had was to put her on high-dose, powerful acid blockers, which she had been taking for years. You will learn in subsequent chapters that acid blockers inhibit your ability to fight infection and your absorption of nutrients.

Jan's struggling immune system caused her to have recurrent throat infections, bronchitis, and pneumonia. Her body was starved for nutrients, manifesting in numbness and muscle weakness that required her to use a cane. The symptoms that were characteristic of MS flared up several times per year, requiring high doses of steroids to suppress an already-dysfunctional immune system.

We partnered to find other ways to reverse her disease. Starting with the basics, we provided her body with immediate nutritional support with a high-quality multivitamin, extra B vitamins, fish oil, and high doses of vitamin D. We supported her gut health with probiotics and digestive enzymes and very slowly started tapering her off the acid blockers reducing the acid that is so important for digestion and absorption of nutrients, as well as preventing infection.

While we supported her nutrition and gut, we started looking for the underlying issues at the root of her disease. We discovered she had a genetic predisposition to celiac disease. Although she tested negative for celiac antibodies, she started a gluten-free diet to help heal her gut. Additional blood tests identified other food triggers that she also eliminated from her diet.

When Jan was a relatively new patient of mine, she read about an interventional procedure to improve blood flow to the brain that was being used to treat patients with MS. After researching it, she found an interventional radiologist at a local university hospital who was performing the procedure on MS patients. Jan had the procedure with my support, and this allowed her to move forward with an unconventional treatment that has been significant to her improvement.

Slowly, over several years, we were able to taper her off the medications, as she no longer needed them. This long period was necessary to alter the course of her disease, but today she takes only three prescription medications. She is no longer on the immune-suppressing drugs for MS. The bloating and constipation are largely gone, and she hasn't had any new MS symptoms in several years.

Most importantly, she no longer uses a cane and still lives in the house she loves. Jan now sees her "disease" in an entirely different way. She appreciates that MS is only a label based on a constellation of symptoms and clinical findings. She considers herself as a person with MS in that sense, but she has discovered that the "disease" is not the same as the cause. By addressing the cause and using the right medical approach, she was able to control her disease and alter its course.

The Solution

Most chronic disease, whether heart disease, high blood pressure, diabetes, Alzheimer's disease, osteoporosis, autoimmune disease, or cancer, has a similar root cause—an imbalance that slowly damages the body. The imbalance leading to disease is a complex interplay of genetics and environment. It starts with certain predisposing factors, such as our genes—whether our mom was healthy when she was pregnant with us, whether we were breastfed or not, early use of antibiotics, and food sensitivities during childhood. Then there are lifestyle factors that set us up for disease, such as processed foods, a sedentary lifestyle, lack of sleep, smoking, and stress. All of these factors create the "perfect storm" that sets the stage for disease. The specific disease we develop is a result of our genetics combined with environmental factors and the lifestyle choices we make.

Functional Medicine is a new approach paving the way for the future of medicine. This philosophy of medicine focuses on identifying the root cause of disease and fixing the imbalance, as opposed to the disease-model approach that matches a medication with the disease. Functional Medicine is a new specialty of medicine that is not organ-specific, but patient-specific. Its approach is unique to each individual—to their genetics as well as their lifestyle. Its focus is to heal and prevent disease with a combination of fuel, movement, rest, and relaxation that will restore the body's powerful natural ability to heal.

The three main components of a Functional Medicine approach—nutrition, exercise, and rest/relaxation—are the strongest and best treatments available, more powerful than any drug that has been or will be developed. This book will show you how almost all chronic disease can be treated, and sometimes cured, by those three components.

Wherever you are on your health journey, this book can help you—whether you're healthy and want to stay healthy, if you have symptoms of an imbalance but haven't yet been diagnosed with a disease, or if you have been labeled with a multitude of diseases and are taking a long list of medications and want to get better.

Although I can give you the information you need, achieving better health is a personal choice, one that you make every day with every decision—whether to eat the cookies that your co-worker brought to work, to go through the drive-through of a fast-food restaurant because you didn't take the time to bring your lunch, to skip the gym today, or to stay up late watching your favorite TV show. The key is to make many more good choices than bad choices.

So, what is your choice going to be? Will you be taking the road toward health, or the one toward disease?

I recommend reading through the book once to get an overview of the material. Then work on the steps you feel comfortable with. Work on each component for one to four weeks. Pay attention to how you feel with each change you make. Find a partner to work with and hold each other accountable.

This book will educate, motivate, and empower you to make simple changes toward better health and well-being. It gives you the resources to make better decisions and show you how to easily implement these habits into your daily life. If you follow the steps in this book, you will alter your course and change your future health destination.

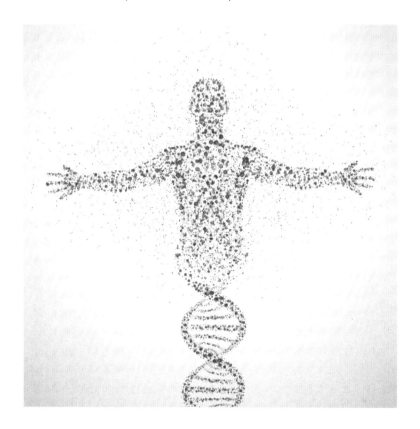

CHAPTER TWO

YOUR GENES ARE NOT YOUR DESTINY

Genes load the gun but environment pulls the trigger.
~ Dr. Francis Collins, Director of National Institutes of Health

A New Perspective on Genes & Disease

People tend to overestimate the contribution that genetics has on their health destiny. So often I hear, "Everyone in my family has diabetes, so I will probably get it." Even in medicine, until recently we thought that genetics was a fixed part of our DNA. However, current findings show that our genes are turned on and off by lifestyle factors.

Food, in particular, plays a large role in whether your genes are expressed or not. Genes contribute only about 20 percent to our health destiny—only a small part of the picture—and the other 80 percent is determined by your lifestyle.[8] Food, movement, sleep, and stress all affect the expression of your genes. Our DNA code is like computer hardware, where our lifestyle choices are the software or operating system that is installed.

Our individual genetics may play a role in determining which disease will surface if our system is out of balance. For example, I might have a genetic predisposition to diabetes and heart disease, so if my system is out of balance, those are the diseases I will develop. You might have a genetic predisposition to autoimmune disease, so when your system is out of balance, you develop an autoimmune disease, such as rheumatoid arthritis or lupus. All of these diseases can be prevented and sometimes even treated through lifestyle changes that, in a sense, switch the genes off.

The trick is catching the imbalance before it becomes a disease. The approach in conventional medicine is to wait for the disease to occur before taking any action. For example, over and over I hear the story of the patient who goes to see their doctor with complaints such as joint pain, headaches, fatigue, or "just not feeling right." They have basic blood tests and are told that nothing is wrong. The patient leaves, thinking, "Maybe it's all in my head." The imbalance continues and the symptoms progress. Time passes and they feel worse and return for another visit. Now that the imbalance is more severe, some abnormalities start to show on blood tests. They finally fit the criteria of a disease that can be matched to a specific drug to mask or reduce symptoms. All the while, nothing has been done to correct the underlying imbalance that triggered the disease in the first place.

Symptoms are your body's way of telling you that things aren't right with the system. To prevent disease, we must approach it using an "upstream" avenue—when you take action at the first sign of imbalance. "Downstream" is when you wait for the disease to develop and then take action. In my experience, the more downstream you start, the harder an imbalance is to correct. It is possible, but takes more time to reverse the imbalance.

Reversing an Incurable Disease

Alzheimer's disease is one of the most devastating and most feared diseases, with no effective treatment and no cure. It robs your memory and your mind and turns your family into caregivers. Alzheimer's disease is a billion-dollar business for the pharmaceutical industry despite the fact that medications are not effective at preventing or treating the disease. By 2050, it is estimated that 160 million people will suffer from Alzheimer's disease.[9] Will you be one of them?

Ten patients were recruited by UCLA researchers to investigate whether lifestyle changes were an effective treatment for Alzheimer's disease. An impressive nine out of ten patients had a reversal of their symptoms, and out of the six who had been forced to leave work because of their diagnosis, all six were able to return to work.[10]

Although this was a small study, the results are remarkable. The protocol included a whole-food, plant-based diet; supplementation with

B vitamins, fish oil, and vitamin D; fasting at least 12 hours between dinner and breakfast; 150 minutes per week of exercise (20 minutes a day); relaxation with yoga, meditation or music; and eight hours of sleep.

The results of this study should have been on the front page of every newspaper or news website, but sadly, it got little press. If a newly discovered drug for Alzheimer's was 90 percent effective, do you think we would hear about it? But lifestyle changes don't sell, and they certainly don't make the headlines.

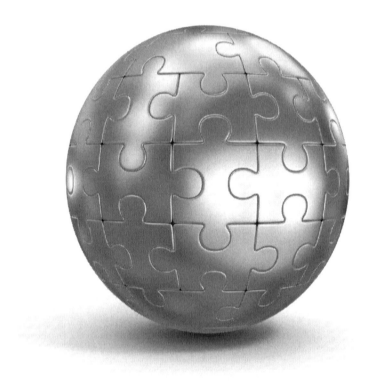

CHAPTER THREE

FIXING DISEASE AT THE ROOT

The part can never be well unless the whole is well.

~ Plato

A different approach is desperately needed to change the direction of Americans' health. Conventional medicine waits for the patient to get sick and then treats them with drugs—most of which block the body's natural ability to function and heal. This strategy is not working. We are getting sicker and sicker with more and more chronic diseases such as diabetes, cancer, heart disease, allergies, asthma, autoimmune disease, osteoporosis, and dementia—all increasing at alarming rates. Drugs are not making us well. We need to make ourselves well!

The goal of a Functional Medicine physician is to work toward restoring and optimizing the incredible power of the body to heal. Symptoms are simply a signal from the body that something is out of balance. The correct approach is to find out why the system is out of balance and restore that balance. We can't reverse the trend of the chronic disease epidemic until we change our approach.

Functional Medicine addresses the underlying causes of disease and considers the patient and physician to be collaborating partners. By shifting from a disease-centered focus to a patient-centered focus, Functional Medicine addresses the person as an individual. It is the future of medicine—and the answer we desperately need.

In the insurance-driven world of conventional medicine, patient encounters have been compressed to woefully inadequate 10- or 15-minute snippets of time. Functional Medicine physicians spend much more time with their patients, listening to their story and considering all the factors influencing health. How to find a Functional Medicine physician is described in the Resources section of this book.

Ty's Story

Ty came to me out of desperation. He was close to losing his job because he couldn't function. He hid in his office, holding his head in his hands, enveloped in severe, debilitating fatigue. He couldn't concentrate or think coherently. Any type of exertion, mental or physical, resulted in a "crash" of exhaustion afterward. He suffered from night sweats, irritability, and body aches, and easily picked up any cold or flu going around. He was afraid to travel. His mysterious illness was not only affecting him, but also his career and, more importantly, his family.

After each visit with many different doctors, he was told his lab values all looked normal. He left the last doctor's office with a referral to a psychologist. Motivated to get better, he agreed to psychotherapy and medications for presumed depression and anxiety. These drugs only made him feel worse.

Chronic Fatigue Syndrome (CFS), or Myalgic Encephalitis (ME), is not a disease, but a constellation of symptoms whose cause is yet to be determined. CFS/ME is the mystery disease of the century. Many different sources have been hypothesized and various infections have been implicated—Epstein Barr Virus, mold infection, a newly discovered virus called XMV. Some researchers theorize patients have a dysfunction of the mitochondria, the part of the cell that produces energy. Most recently, scientists have postulated that the cause lies in a heightened sensitivity of the nerves and have a new name for CFS/ME—neuromuscular central sensitivity. Because CFS/ME has no known source, most doctors

Stacey J. Robinson, MD

me it's not real—that CFS is a psychological problem.
he only offered treatments are anti-depressant
and psychotherapy.

Since the goal is to look for imbalances in the system and correct them, we examined Ty's diet first. He had nutritional deficiencies that were corrected with food and supplements. He wasn't sleeping, so we focused on getting him adequate rest through changes in lifestyle, supplements, and some initial medications. He cut down on processed carbohydrates and sugars, which Ty's fatigued body was craving for quick energy.

We also detected a genetic abnormality in his body's ability to activate folate, an important nutrient that helps the body detoxify, so we supplemented with the activated form of that vitamin. About 15 percent of the population has a significant abnormality in this folate-activating enzyme, called MTHFR, causing the body to have an impaired ability in removing environmental toxins.

Ty cleaned up his diet in order to reduce exposure to those toxins. He also increased his intake of organic vegetables and fruits through blending and juicing which provides nutrients that assist the body's detoxification process. We also corrected hormone deficiencies common in CFS/ME with hormone replacement.

When he started feeling better, he was able to slowly get back into exercising. After a year or two, Ty was off all drugs. Although he occasionally has symptoms if he doesn't keep his healthy lifestyle in check, he is 95 percent better. His career is successful and he is doing things he hasn't done in years, like traveling and surfing. Finally, Ty can spend quality time with his family.

Road Map to Health: 7 Steps to Alter Your Destination

PART II—THE SEVEN STEPS

28

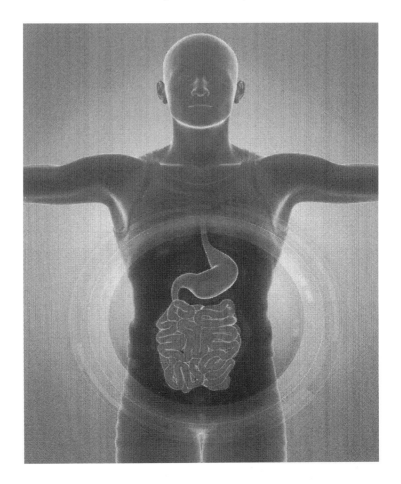

CHAPTER FOUR

STEP ONE: FIX YOUR GUT

All disease begins in the gut.

~ Hippocrates

To quote Rodney Dangerfield, "I don't get no respect . . ." and neither does the gut! While the gut is definitely the least appreciated organ in the body, it is probably the root cause of most chronic disease. Patients don't like to talk about the gut because it is embarrassing. Symptoms like bloating, flatulence, constipation, diarrhea, and changes in stool are not pleasant conversations, even at doctor visits. But the gut is really the center of your body's universe, and if your gut isn't healthy, you won't be, either. It is difficult to comprehend how inflammation in the gut can affect distant organs like the heart, brain, or skin, but the gut has far-reaching effects, as you will learn in this chapter.

Poor gut health is associated with diseases inside the gut, such as irritable bowel syndrome (IBS), esophageal disorders, and inflammatory bowel diseases. However, most people don't realize that poor gut health is associated with many diseases outside of the gut, including osteoporosis; allergies and asthma; neurological diseases, including depression, anxiety, dementia, and attention deficient disorder; autoimmune disease, such as lupus, rheumatoid arthritis, and thyroid disease; and even skin diseases such as eczema, rosacea, psoriasis, and acne.

The Gut Does a Whole Lot More than You Think

Your gut is basically an open tube, from mouth to anus, and is technically outside your body, since this surface area has direct communication with the outside environment. The gut is the largest barrier between you and the outside world and is approximately 16 feet long and lined with fingerlike projections called "villi." If you were to stretch out your gut and all those villi, the surface area would cover about 350 square feet, or the size of a small studio apartment![11]

Your gut has the very important job of bringing in what your body needs and keeping out what it doesn't. When that doesn't happen, your health will suffer. The following are the critical functions that your gut must perform to keep you healthy.

Letting in the Good—The average person eats almost a ton of food per year. From that ton that passes through, the gut has a very complex process of identifying and filtering those nutrients you need and allowing for their absorption into the blood stream. The effectiveness of this absorption process is determined by the integrity of the gut's surface area. You probably appreciate that your gut is where you digest and absorb food, but that's just the beginning.

Identifying the Enemy—Food entering your body also contains chemicals and pathogens (viruses, bacteria, and parasites) that shouldn't gain entry. Because the gut is your first line of defense against these toxins and infection, 70 percent of your immune system resides within your gut, called the Gut Associated Lymphoid Tissue.[12] So it makes sense that diseases associated with imbalance of the immune system, such as allergies, asthma, and autoimmune diseases, have their origins in an unhealthy gut. These diseases are heavily on the rise.

Taking Out the Garbage—The gut is the primary center of your body's detoxification system, which is simply your body's way of eliminating the toxins you are exposed to every day. The gut plays many roles in detoxification, including identifying and filtering pathogens and chemicals, receiving toxic by-products from the liver, and eliminating this waste via bowel movements. The good bacteria that live in your gut also help detoxify the chemicals you ingest. You will learn much more about these friendly bacteria later in this chapter.

The Second Brain—The gut produces 70–80 percent of your body's serotonin, the neurotransmitter that positively influences your mood and sense of well-being.[13] The gut has been called "the second brain" because it's rich in other neurotransmitters, too—the chemicals your brain uses to communicate with the rest of your body. This allows an interconnection between the gut and the brain; however, most of the conversation goes from the gut to the brain, rather than the other way around. There is evidence that the good bacteria in your gut actually communicates with the brain via the vagus nerve that connects them.[14]

If your gut is not healthy, your brain isn't going to be healthy, either. Some of the neurological symptoms occurring from poor gut health include brain fog, difficulty concentrating, anxiety, and depression.

In our "pill for every ill" approach, doctors tend to reach for their prescription pad. American physicians' plan of attack to fix depression is to prescribe medications that increase levels of serotonin. This class of medications, referred to as Selective Serotonin Reuptake Inhibitors (SSRIs), include Prozac, Zoloft, and Paxil, among others. In some studies, they demonstrate a modest improvement of depression, but other studies show no effect at all over a placebo. The bottom line is that these medications do not address the underlying cause and have significant side effects. Topping the list, not surprisingly, are gastrointestinal symptoms.

Eight Reasons Why Your Gut Might Not Be Healthy

So, where did we go wrong? Why do we have an epidemic of disease that has poor gut health as its root cause?

1) Toxic Load—In the United States, over 10,000 chemicals are added to the food supply. Eighty-percent of these lack adequate safety studies.[15] These chemicals can damage the lining of the gut and kill the good bacteria that keep your gut healthy and help your body to absorb nutrients and detoxify.[16,17]

One of the most important actions you can take for better health is to "eat clean" in order to reduce your exposure to these chemicals. We will go into detail about how to eat a clean diet in Chapters 4 and 5.

2) Lack of "Good Bugs"—In order to stay healthy, your gut needs a community of friendly bacteria that outnumber your body's cells by a ratio of about 10:1. You have ten trillion cells in your body, but a healthy body should have 100 trillion organisms in it, and most of them live in your gut.

These "good bugs," also called probiotics, are collectively called the "microbiome" or "body flora." This community of friendly bacteria has many roles, including digestion and absorption of nutrients, vitamin production, and preventing bad bacteria, viruses, and parasites from taking up residence. Probiotics also decrease inflammation, which is the common factor in almost all chronic disease.

The complex and powerful role of the microbiome is a topic of study in its infancy. We are just starting to understand its powerful role in health and disease. More and more evidence supports the idea that the lack of a healthy microbiome is at the root of a variety of diseases, including depression, anxiety, autism, Parkinson's disease, obesity, diabetes, rheumatoid arthritis, IBS, and ulcerative colitis.

Why is a lack of this healthy microbiome so pervasive? There are multiple reasons. First, we live in a germaphobic world filled with hand sanitizer in every home, store, school, purse, and backpack. Our food comes out of a factory, sterilized and clean. We no longer preserve our food through fermentation (which adds good bacteria) because we have chemical preservatives that keep food on the shelf for years. And the many drugs and chemicals which you are exposed to alter the microbiome, including antibiotics and acid blockers, and artificial sweeteners, preservatives, and other chemicals in food.

The pervasive use of unnecessary antibiotics is an enormous contributor to an unhealthy gut and the epidemic of chronic disease. Additionally, the food you eat—or don't eat—alters the balance of bacteria in your gut. You will learn more about the foods that support or inhibit a healthy microbiome in Chapter 5.

3) Lack of Fiber—The average American eats about 15 grams of fiber, which is only half of the 30 or so grams needed for a healthy gut.[18] We don't get enough fiber because we don't eat enough plant foods like vegetables, fruits, nuts, seeds, and legumes. Fiber provides food for our microbiome and also keeps bowel movements regular.

4) Chronic Constipation—Almost 20 percent of the population suffers from chronic constipation.[19] Bowel movements are the final step in eliminating toxins from your body. Contributing to this elimination problem are a diet lacking in fiber, inadequate water intake, a sedentary lifestyle, and a lack of nutrients such as magnesium. Slow transit time through the intestines allows toxins more time to be absorbed into the system.

5) Damage to the Lining of the Gut—When the barrier function of the gut is damaged, we call that an increase in intestinal permeability, or a "leaky gut." When this happens, toxins, pathogens, and larger food particles can move into the blood stream and cause our immune system—which produces antibodies against these "intruders"—to react. Antibodies are proteins that attach and neutralize the intruders. When the gut is leaky and the immune system is producing an array of antibodies, the antibodies can mistakenly identify our own body tissue as the intruder and trigger an autoimmune disease.

Although autoimmune disease is classified and treated by specialists based on the organ system involved, there is evidence that all autoimmune disease has its root in abnormal intestinal permeability.[20, 21, 22] Healing the gut is the most important component of preventing and treating autoimmune disease.

6) Medications—Many drugs can wreak havoc on the gut. Non-steroidal anti-inflammatory drugs (NSAIDS) are one of the biggest offenders. Many of these are available over the counter, like ibuprofen (Advil) and naproxen (Aleve), and are taken by millions of people without any knowledge of their effects on gut health.

Another enormous problem is acid blockers, used to reduce the symptoms of heartburn and also available without a prescription. They have many deleterious effects on gut function by reducing the acidic environment essential to protein digestion and immune function. The acidic environment in our stomach is the first line of defense to kill pathogens. This is why people who take acid blockers have an increased risk of gastrointestinal infections and pneumonia.[23, 24]

7) Food Sensitivities—Gluten (a protein found in wheat, barley, and rye) damages the lining of the gut in some people. Other foods that can cause sensitivity and damage to the gut's lining include soy, dairy, corn, eggs, and nuts.

8) Stress—Stress also increases gut permeability, which may be why high levels of stress are frequently a trigger of disease, especially autoimmune disease. Patients often report that they felt fine until a stressful event that preceded the disease process. You will learn much more about how stress causes disease in Chapter 6.

Angelica's Story

Angelica is an 18-year-old young lady who came to see me in 2014, a year after she was diagnosed with rheumatoid arthritis at the age of 16. Her parents brought her in for a second opinion and were looking for a Functional Medicine approach to her disease.

Prior to her diagnosis, she considered herself healthy, except for allergies and asthma. As a young child, she had recurrent throat and respiratory infections that led to her being treated with antibiotics many times. She also fractured her left wrist at age seven, which later was the joint that the rheumatoid arthritis settled in.

In March of 2013, she started having mild, intermittent stiffness in her fingers. By October of the same year, she had pain and stiffness in her shoulders and ankles, her left wrist swelled up, and she could barely walk. At that time, blood tests showed some inflammation, but tests for rheumatoid arthritis were negative. It wasn't until April of 2014 that her blood tests became positive for rheumatoid arthritis. Two years after she started having symptoms, she finally could be "labeled" with a disease, but by that time, she had severe bone erosion in her wrist. She then saw a rheumatologist and was started on very powerful medications to suppress her immune system and slow the damage to her joints.

Because there is an association between celiac disease and other autoimmune conditions, I tested Angelica to see if it might have been a predisposing factor to her developing rheumatoid arthritis. Celiac disease is usually not suspected in the absence of the classic symptoms, such as weight loss and diarrhea, described in medical textbooks. However, about 30 percent of patients with celiac disease do not have classic symptoms, and some have no symptoms at all [25]. Everyone with an autoimmune condition should be tested for celiac disease.

It turned out that Angelica did have celiac disease, likely to be the root cause of her rheumatoid arthritis. Upon further questioning, she had a history of chronic constipation and some food allergies. The frequent antibiotics during her childhood probably contributed to an imbalance in her gut that set her up for the disease.

Although we initially decided to keep Angelica on the immune-suppressing drugs to prevent further joint destruction, the most important components of Angelica's treatment were to put her on a strict gluten-free diet, remove other food triggers, and add additional *nutrients to heal her gut. After 12 months of treatment, she felt almost 100 percent better. Her allergies and asthma improved. She even had some reversal of the joint destruction in her wrist.*

The best part of the story is that Angelica's goal now is to become a physician and specialize in rheumatology, helping other patients through a similar approach to autoimmune diseases.

Six Steps to a Healthy Gut

1) Eat a Clean Diet—One of the most important steps you can take toward better health is to decrease your exposure to chemicals that damage the gut. Eating a clean diet means one free of chemicals and other added ingredients such as pesticides, artificial sweeteners, preservatives, GMOs, hormones, antibiotics, heavy metals, BPA, and phthalates. The details and simple tools to eat a clean diet are given in Chapter 5.

2) Avoid Medications that Impair Gut Function—Unless absolutely necessary, avoid anti-inflammatory pain medications (NSAIDS), acid blockers (H_2 Blockers and Proton Pump Inhibitors), steroids, and antibiotics.

3) Eat Foods that Support the Microbiome— Probiotic-rich foods do just that. We all know yogurt has probiotics, but it's important to eat a variety of foods containing them, as well as to eat foods that contain prebiotics. Those foods are composed of certain plant fibers that provide food for the good bacteria (more on this in Chapter 5).

4) Eliminate Trigger Foods—Certain foods can contribute to poor gut health, either by damaging the lining of the gut or by promoting inflammation. People who have an unhealthy gut tend to react to these foods. As mentioned, common triggers include gluten, dairy, soy, corn, eggs, nuts, citrus, and nightshades. Eliminating these foods for four weeks can give the body a break and allow the gut to heal.

After the healing time, reintroduce one food every week to see if you experience any symptoms. Common physical warnings of food intolerance include bloating, nausea, diarrhea, brain fog, joint pain, headache, or fatigue.

5) Reduce Stress—Spend at least 15 minutes per day relaxing. Relaxation is essential to healing and maintaining gut health. See Chapter 6 for more on stress reduction.

6) Get Help with Supplements—Consider adding supplements that promote gut healing, such as probiotics, omega-3 essential fatty acids, digestive enzymes, zinc, magnesium, and L-Glutamine. I recommend finding a Functional Medicine practitioner to help guide you with this component.

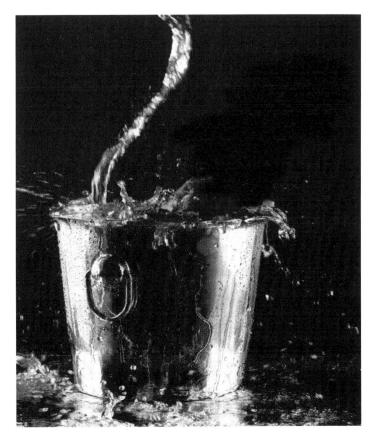

CHAPTER FIVE

STEP TWO: EMPTY THE BUCKET

Take care of your body. It's the only place you have to live.

~ Jim Rohn

One of the most misused and misunderstood words in the world of health and fitness is "detoxification." Detoxification is not a colon cleansing kit purchased at the drugstore, nor a colon flush from your local colon therapist, nor a foot bath that turns a different color because toxins are professed to be coming out of your feet. And it is not simply a 3-, 7-, or 14-day juice fast.

Detoxification is something your body does naturally every moment of every day in order to rid your body of the waste it produces and the toxins it accumulates from your environment. The complexity of this process is nothing short of amazing. Theodor Herzl, a poet, playwright, and journalist, described it beautifully when he said, "The body is a marvelous machine... a chemical laboratory, a power-house. Every movement, voluntary or involuntary, full of secrets and marvels!"[26]

Without our innate detoxification mechanisms, we would die. To do its job, your body requires many components to carry out the function of "cleaning house." The primary organs of detoxification are the liver, kidneys, lymphatic system, and gastrointestinal tract. While detoxification is something your body normally accomplishes, it does require specific nutrients and substrates to do the job, and it also requires the organs involved to function optimally.

Although you won't find a list of symptoms for "impaired detoxification" in medical textbooks, we do see a characteristic set of symptoms in those whose "bucket runneth over." These symptoms include—but are not limited to—fatigue, headache, muscle and joint pain, bloating, sinus congestion and allergies, skin rashes and acne, anxiety, depression, brain fog, and weight gain.

In clinical practice, addressing this constellation of symptoms by reducing chemical exposure and supporting the body's detoxification system results in symptom improvement and in reduction in blood inflammatory markers.

Seven Essential Components of Detoxification

1) Reduce Exposure—There are multiple strategies and tools that can help you reduce your exposure to chemicals in the environment. You will learn about them in detail in Chapter 5.

2) Nutrients—For detoxification to work properly, our liver needs over 25 nutrients to help it transform toxins and prepare them for elimination. You will hear more about what foods provide these nutrients in Chapter 5. If you aren't eating foods that are high in these nutrients, your liver is not going to be as efficient at detoxification. In addition, some genetic abnormalities slow the detoxification system, which may predispose you to diseases of impaired detoxification such as cancer and autoimmune disease. Using a garbage analogy, the liver puts the trash inside the garbage can, getting it ready for disposal.

3) Movement—The lymphatic system, like the circulatory system, is a network of vessels that carry fluid around the body. Its job is to filter waste and carry it out of our system. The lymphatic system carries pathogens, toxins, and waste to the lymph nodes, spleen, and thymus. These act as filters, allowing our immune system to identify and remove them. Unlike the circulatory system, the lymphatic system does not have a pump like the heart, requiring body movement to move the filtered fluid throughout your anatomy.

Since it moves toxins by way of muscle and joint contractions, a sedentary lifestyle, in which we sit and work for the majority of our day, hampers the lymphatic system from moving and filtering these toxins. Other ways that the lymphatics move fluid is through massage, as well as breathing movements of our chest wall. Again using the garbage analogy, the lymphatic system carries all the trash from around the house and brings it to a central location.

4) Bowel Movements—Elimination of stool needs to be regular because that's how those accumulated toxins are removed from the gut. Again using our garbage analogy, bowel movements are equivalent to the garbage man coming to take the trash away from our house.

In order to eliminate properly, our gut needs fiber, water, movement, relaxation, and a healthy microbiome. You should have at the very least one bowel movement a day; however, given a proper diet, bowel movements two or three times per day is probably reflective of a healthier diet, gut and detoxification process.

5) Water—Your body is 60 percent water, all of your cells are bathed in water, and your kidneys need water to flush out your system. Water is like a rinse for the entire body. It's analogous to washing out all the dirty garbage cans that you just emptied. Are you neglecting this essential component that helps your body stay healthy?

6) Sleep—Your body does much of its repair work while you sleep. It is so important to have adequate sleep to give your body the time to repair. Evidence shows sleep is literally a detox for the brain. Researchers confirmed for the first time that the space between cells increases during sleep, allowing the brain to flush out toxins that build up during waking hours.[27] Read more about the healing power of sleep in Chapter 7.

7) Reduce Stress—The detoxification process is impaired by stress in a multitude of ways. Stress promotes inflammation, which creates additional internal waste that needs to be eliminated. Stress promotes constipation, a leaky gut, and an imbalanced microbiome. It makes us crave junk food, which adds toxicity from processed foods. We also sleep and exercise less when we are under stress.

"Your Bucket Runneth Over"

I like to use the bucket analogy because I think it is a simple way to understand what happens when the detoxification process is overwhelmed, and how that fits in with symptoms and disease. Every toxin you are exposed to adds to filling the bucket, and our detoxification process is the way we empty the bucket. When the bucket overflows, you don't feel well. If the bucket continues to overflow, you will eventually develop chronic disease. The toxins filling the bucket are many—air pollution and cigarette smoke; environmental chemicals in tap and bottled water, cosmetics, cleaners, air fresheners, and food containers; and chemicals in processed foods, including additives and preservatives, artificial sweeteners, nitrates, pesticides, trans-fats, hormones, and antibiotics.

To empty the bucket, you need nutrients to fuel your liver, normal bowel movements, a healthy microbiome, clean water to flush out your system, muscle movement to get the lymphatics flowing, and sleep/relaxation so that your body has time to repair and recover.

Underlying this inflow and outflow of toxins are some issues with our genetic predisposition for efficient detoxification, as mentioned above. Many people have genetic SNPs (single nucleotide polymorphisms), which are abnormalities in the genetic code that control the production of detoxification enzymes. Enzymes are proteins that help these detoxification processes occur more rapidly. Genetic SNP abnormalities can result in decreased enzyme production.

The most commonly known SNP is for the MTHFR gene, an enzyme that activates folate, a B vitamin necessary for the liver detoxification pathway. If you have an MTHFR SNP, you have a reduced capacity to produce that enzyme, and may have impaired detoxification. People with MTHFR SNPs have increased risk of heart disease, psychiatric disorders, and Parkinson's disease.[28,29,30] The MTHFR SNP can be identified by a simple blood test. If you have this SNP, you may benefit from taking the activated form of folate and other B-vitamins to support the detoxification pathway.

Inflammation

When detoxification is impaired, a chronic, smoldering inflammation occurs. We are all familiar with acute inflammation. When we have an illness or injury, the body reacts by producing heat, redness, swelling, and pain. Inflammation is a very complex cascade of events put into action by our immune system. This acute type of inflammation is good because it helps the body protect itself and heal from the injury.

On the other hand, inflammation that occurs when our bucket overflows—either due to too many toxins, impaired detoxification, or both—is hidden and silent. This is referred to as "chronic inflammation" and increases the incidence of all chronic disease, including cancer, heart disease, diabetes, osteoporosis, asthma, allergies, autoimmune disease, dementia, and skin diseases. This internal inflammation can't always be seen; however, we can detect it with blood tests—most commonly, a test called hsCRP. Inflammation is a sign of imbalance. Some people have symptoms related to inflammation, such as fluid retention, headaches, joint pain, brain fog, or fatigue.

Inflammation increases your risk of cancer by 47 to 82 percent, and also increases the risk of death from cancer and increases the risk that cancer will recur.[31] Cancer may, in fact, be a disease of impaired detoxification. An estimated minimum of 30 percent of cancer cases are linked to our diet, processed foods, and a lack of nutrient-rich food.[32]

It is unfortunate that conventional medicine doesn't embrace nutrition as a prevention tool. We spend over $5 billion per year on cancer research, with less than 6 percent of that money going toward prevention.[33]

Stephanie's Story

Stephanie came into my office to establish care. She reported a history of constipation "all her life" and migraines since age 12. Happily married and wanting desperately to have a child, she and her husband had seen many infertility specialists and suffered through five miscarriages. She had recently been diagnosed with autoimmune thyroid disease.

Despite her thyroid labs being "normal," she did not feel well and reported headaches, "brain fog," weight gain, and fatigue. Initial testing was positive for celiac disease and Stephanie had a very high hsCRP, a sign of inflammation. She also was positive for the MTHFR mutation, indicating an impaired ability to activate folate, an important nutrient for the detoxification pathway. In addition, her cholesterol was very high and her blood sugar level was elevated—in the pre-diabetes range.

The focus for Stephanie was to be on a strict gluten-free diet and to reduce her exposure to chemicals with a clean diet. We also switched her to a thyroid medication that was guaranteed gluten free. It's ironic that while there is a strong connection between celiac and thyroid disease, the most common thyroid medications are not guaranteed to be free of gluten. We also checked all of her supplements to make sure they were gluten free. Many inactive ingredients in supplements and medications come from wheat and therefore contain gluten. We worked on getting her bowels moving better with fiber, herbals, magnesium, and probiotics. She also addressed other food sensitivities—detected by additional blood testing—by cutting those foods out of her diet.

After only three months, she was feeling better and her hsCRP was reduced by half. Her cholesterol and cardiac risk markers were reduced to almost normal levels and her blood sugar levels were no longer in the pre-diabetic range. Within a year, she had also lost 30 pounds. This result was simply achieved with changes in her diet and supplements to support her own body's healing mechanisms.

The Biggest Enemy—Chemicals in Our Environment

Our biggest detoxification issues come from the 84,000 chemicals on the market today used in food, personal care and household products. Of these products that we come in contact with every day, only about 1 percent of these have been studied for safety.[34] As mentioned earlier, only 20% of the chemicals used in food processing have safety studies. Even more frightening, only 7% have been tested for safety in pregnancy and childhood development.[35] Often it is not until after these chemicals are found to be harmful that they are removed from our food supply—sometimes decades after they were introduced. When this data was presented at the 2010 hearing of the Senate Subcommittee on Superfund, Toxics and Environmental Health, Senator Frank Lautenberg told the committee that such little oversight means that children in the United States are virtual "guinea pigs in an uncontrolled experiment".

Take trans-fats, for example. These chemically altered fats were created in the 1970s to make fats solid at room temperature—so consumers could have a spreadable margarine to put on their toast. Here we are, four decades later, removing trans-fats from our foods because now we know these chemically altered fats cause disease. We are all guinea pigs for the food industry.

Another example of how food safety can be misleading is the "Generally Regarded as Safe" (GRAS) designation. Chemicals that have been tested and found to be safe in small amounts are categorized as GRAS; however, these may not be safe in larger amounts, or when combined with other chemicals. For example, the safety of artificial sweeteners—including Sweet'n Low, Splenda, NutraSweet, and Equal—have been in question for decades. Most people assume they are safe because they are allowed in our food supply. There may be animal studies demonstrating safety in small amounts; however, many people consume large amounts of these sweeteners.

If you drink a 12-pack of diet sodas per day, you're probably taking in a much higher amount than the amount approved for safe ingestion. Or if you are eating a variety of "no sugar added" or "diet" foods, you are getting artificial sweeteners in multiple food sources. Many people are taking in much more than what may be a "safe" amount, and no one is even considering how these thousands of chemicals being consumed may interact together to cause disease.

A 2015 analysis published in the cancer journal, *Carcinogenesis*, suggests that there is, in fact, a cumulative effect of chemicals that promotes the development of cancer and that chemical exposure from our food and environment may contribute to as much as 19 percent of cancers.[36] This is very concerning for our health future, especially given the increasing number of chemicals in our environment.

Chemicals in food packaging materials are also another significant source of toxins, particularly a class of chemicals called endocrine-disrupting chemicals (EDCs). EDCs mimic the hormones in our body. One of the biggest categories is that of Bisphenol A (BPA), a chemical used to make plastics and lining of cans. You will learn more about how to avoid BPA in the next chapter.

One of the most important actions you can take for better health is to learn how to reduce the number of chemicals you ingest. We will cover this in detail in the next chapter.

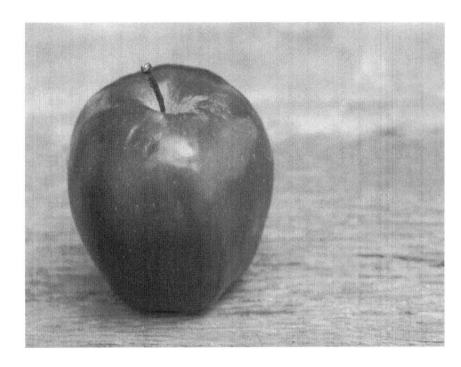

CHAPTER SIX

STEP THREE: FUEL YOUR BODY WITH REAL FOOD

The food you eat can be either the safest and most powerful form of medicine or the slowest form of poison.

~ Ann Wigmore

Humans have known for thousands of years that food is one of the most important components of our health. Hippocrates, known as the "Father of Western Medicine", was quoted as saying "Let food be thy medicine, and medicine be thy food" around 300 B.C. Unfortunately, the "Western Medicine" that he founded has strayed far from this premise. Processed food is not real food. It is a manufactured food-like substance made from some real food components plus added salt, sugar, flavors, colors, and chemicals that alter its appearance, improve the shelf life, and make us crave it. It's a reconstructed food, put together in a box, bag, can, or microwave-ready meal. With the advent of processed foods, we have become disconnected from the origin and definition of real, whole foods. Worse, we're raising a society of people who don't know how to cook—other than heating up a ready-to-go meal.

Four Ways to Connect with Food

1) Think of Food as Fuel. We need to become more connected with food, thinking of it as fuel and as building blocks for our body. We literally become what we eat. The nutrients gained from food are converted into our body structure and function. It's estimated that we build a whole new skeleton in seven to ten years.[37] Where does that skeleton come from? It comes from the nutrients we eat and our body's ability to make living tissue.

The fact that you can change what you eat and then change the structure of your body is something people usually don't think about. Many consider food as only calories that come from protein, carbohydrates and fat, but the fact that food literally becomes us is not appreciated. Nutrient-rich foods help us to thrive, while processed foods can lead to a slow death.

2) Eat Real Food. There is a well-known saying by food activist Michael

Pollan: "Don't eat anything that your great-grandmother wouldn't recognize as food."[38] Examples of real and whole food include fresh fruits and vegetables, beans, whole grains, nuts and seeds, eggs, seafood, and meats (from the butcher, not the deli).

3) Help Your Body Digest. Digestion starts in the brain and involves all our senses. It starts when you engage your brain by thinking about food, smelling it while it is cooking, and admiring a delicious meal. In response, your brain prepares your body for digestion, releasing hormones and digestive enzymes that will break down the food into absorbable nutrients. The digestive process continues in the mouth, with our teeth, grinding up the food, and enzymes in our saliva beginning the breakdown.

Often we eat a pre-made meal, standing up, or in the car and "on the go," and then wonder why we have digestive problems. We don't chew our food slowly or for long enough to allow the digestive process to happen as it should. We inhale our food and then are surprised when we have bloating or heartburn.

4) Slow Down. Meals should be relaxing, not rushed. As much as possible, use mealtime to either spend time alone to reflect, or to enjoy fellowship and connection with friends and family. We're really not giving food the respect it deserves as fuel for both our body as well as our soul.

Food Fight of the Decade

There's always controversy in the media about what is the perfect diet, and it often seems like everyone believes that *their* new fad diet is the best one. Arguments abound for eating in various ways: low-fat, low-carb, high-fat/ketotic, Mediterranean, vegan, and Paleo. The fad diets come in every name, shape, and form. Sadly, we're really losing perspective on the importance of just eating clean, whole foods.

If you follow nutritional gurus in the media and on social media sites, you may have noticed the ongoing battle between those who promote a vegan diet and those who promote a Paleo diet. Vegans believe that animal products and fats cause chronic disease and that a diet high in veggies, fruits, and grains is best. Paleo proponents like their veggies, too, but think that grass-fed and wild meats are important for health. They believe that grains, starches, and sugars are the real health killers.

Results of medical studies can be used to support either side, as the evidence is inconsistent and mostly based on anecdotal and retrospective studies. These studies group carbohydrates, fats, and proteins into categories without considering the quality of the food itself.

We won't know the answer (if there is one) until we have a head-to-head study between Paleo and vegan diets that are both made up of clean, unprocessed foods. It's very likely that processed foods and "food-like" substances not found in nature are the real culprit to our epidemic of chronic disease.

What is obvious is that these two ways of eating have more in common than their differences. Both can be part of a healthy diet. Paleo followers and vegans would probably agree with Michael Pollen, author and food activist, when he said simply, "Eat food. Not too much. Mostly plants."[39] Every day in my practice I'm asked what I think is the healthiest diet. I am a proponent of the diet I call "Eat Real, Clean Food." We are all biochemically unique and there is no one correct diet that works well for everyone. It is important to listen to your body and also watch biochemical markers that indicate your risk of disease to see what type of diet improves those markers.

Both the Paleo and vegan diets can work well and there are positive aspects to both—such as avoiding sugar and eliminating or limiting dairy, not counting calories, and simply eating real food. On a vegan diet, it's important to get adequate protein, vitamin B_{12}, and omega-3 fatty acids, and to avoid too much sugar or processed flour. On a Paleo diet, it is important to avoid factory-farmed meats and only eat clean, sustainable fish. Any meat from an unhealthy animal—one that is fed foods it doesn't eat in nature, injected full of hormones and antibiotics, and/or forced into crowded, cruel, and stressful conditions—is not healthy food.

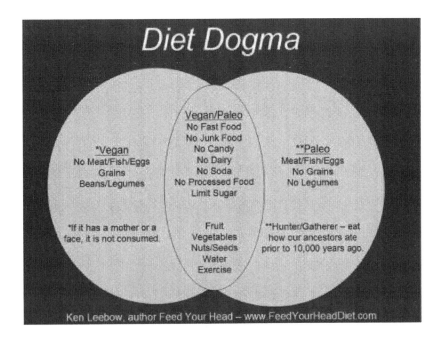

Eight Steps to Eat a Clean Diet

1) Reduce Your Exposure to Pesticides. You can reduce your exposure to pesticides by approximately 80 percent if you buy organic for the foods listed in the Dirty Dozen™. Published annually by the Environmental Working Group (EWG), it lists the produce containing the highest amount of pesticides. Conversely, the Clean Fifteen™ is a list of the produce with the lowest levels of pesticides. You do not need to buy organic for them. You can find this list at EWG.org or download the Dirty Dozen app for your smartphone. See the 2016 EWG guide in Appendix I.

As mentioned before, making sure you are ridding your body of toxins is so important to gut health. Part of that is eliminating—or at least reducing—the number of pesticides and contaminants that you consume. If you don't have access to organic produce, be sure to wash your produce with the following recipe to remove as much pesticide residue as possible.

Homemade Produce Wash to Remove Pesticides

1 cup water

1 cup vinegar

2 tbsp baking soda

2 tsp lemon juice

Mix together, then scrub produce, or let them soak for several minutes before rinsing.

2) Avoid Meats & Dairy from Factory Farms. Animals grown in feedlots for mass production of food are raised in such crowded, unhealthy conditions that they require antibiotics to be free of disease. They are given cheap food lacking in nutrients, like GMO corn and soy (more about GMOs below), and some are injected with hormones to grow faster and fatter. These animals supply the majority of meats, poultry, and fish in our grocery stores and restaurants.

Animals raised in this manner are not healthy, and neither is their flesh. Purchase organic, free-range poultry, eggs, and dairy and grass-fed beef whenever possible.

3) Eat Clean Seafood. The chemicals used to make our lives more convenient have made their way into our water, polluting our fish. And fish aren't immune to the feed-lot phenomenon. Like beef and poultry, some seafood is fished or farmed in harmful ways that make its consumption unhealthy and harmful to your body.

For example, farmed salmon is very unhealthy. The fish are fed corn and soy (because they are inexpensive) and raised in very crowded, stressful conditions. Because the fish are not healthy, they are an unappealing gray color, so their flesh is artificially colored. Many people eat salmon because of its omega-3 content; however, farmed salmon is not high in healthy omega-3 fats, like its wild counterpart, because it isn't raised naturally. In addition, many larger, predatory fish like tuna, shark, and swordfish are high in mercury, which can cause health problems.

There are excellent guides to help you eat sustainable, healthier seafood. The Seafood Selector, created by the Environmental Defense Fund (EDF), advises users in ensuring you are eating the cleanest and most sustainable seafood. By monitoring the type of fish you eat, you can greatly reduce your exposure to chemicals.

The Seafood Selector categorizes seafood as Eco-Best (clean and sustainable), Eco-OK, or Eco-Worst. You can download and print a pocket card to carry with you at seafood.EDF.org. Guides based on specific geographic regions of the world are available, and sushi pocket guides for those who enjoy eating sushi. See the EDF Seafood Selector guide in Appendix II.

If you refer to the guide, you will notice that it isn't necessarily the type of fish that is important, but where and how the fish was caught. When you are eating at a restaurant, don't be afraid to ask about the origin of the fish or shellfish. Another helpful guide, available as a smartphone app, is Seafood Watch, published by the Monterey Bay Aquari

4) Avoid BPA. As mentioned in the last chapter, BPA (Bisphenol A) is a chemical used to make plastics and resins that may contribute to cancer and disrupt your body's hormone function. The following are tips to reduce your exposure to BPA and other EDCs.

- Avoid drinking water from plastic bottles. Drink filtered water from a glass container instead.

- Do not microwave foods in plastic wrap or plastic containers. Use ceramic or glass instead. There is no "microwave safe" plastic.

- Store your food in glass or ceramic containers, wax paper, brown paper bags, or a metal thermos.

- Use wax paper instead of plastic wrap.

- Transfer purchased food that is wrapped in plastic to another container as soon as you return home.

- Keep plastic out of the dishwasher, freezer, and microwave. BPA leaches out of plastic more readily at hot or cold temperatures.

- Avoid plastic containers with numbers 3, 6, and 7 (the recycling number on the bottom of the container). The safest recycling-numbered plastic containers are #1 single use (but do not reuse), 2, 4, and 5. Look for brands that say "PVC free" or "BPA free."

- Avoid canned food and drinks unless the can says it is BPA free. The insides of most cans are lined with BPA.

- Leave your store receipts behind. Most thermal paper used for printed receipts contains BPA.

- Make sure children's toys, baby bottles, pacifiers, and sippy cups are BPA free.

- Make sure your dentist uses BPA-free sealants and composites.

5) Avoid GMO Foods. Genetically modified foods contain genetic material that does not occur in nature or through traditional crossbreeding agricultural methods. Genetic material is inserted into the DNA of a plant or animal to make it behave differently. For example, GMO plants can be made to resist certain pesticides. GMO salmon, approved for consumption in the United States in November 2015, is made to grow twice as fast.[40] The problem is that we don't know how eating these foods may affect our long-term health.

A growing body of evidence links GMO foods with health problems. A recent article in the most respected health journal, the *New England Journal of Medicine*, finally brought the GMO problem to the attention of the medical community and pointed out several very worrisome facts about pesticide-resistant GMO crops. The science supporting safety of GMOs is flawed and has been provided by the pesticide manufacturer, who benefits financially from the widespread use of GMO crops. Since GMO foods were introduced, the use of the pesticide glyphosate, a known carcinogen, has increased by 250 percent. This pesticide has not been determined to be safe for our children. [41]

The National Academy of Sciences has put together a committee to look at the safety of GMOs and the pesticides used on GMO crops, but it will probably take years to come to a conclusion. In the meantime, GMO foods remain unlabeled and ubiquitous in your food, creating one of the largest unregulated experiments ever conducted—with Americans as test subjects, jeopardizing your health and the health of children who are our future.

Most countries do not consider GMOs to be safe and have restrictions or bans on their use. The US government has approved GMOs based on evidence presented by the same corporations that created them and profit from their sale. This enormous, unacceptable conflict of interest puts the safety of your health at risk. American consumers, not having given any consent, are part of this huge GMO safety experiment. The results may not be apparent for decades.

The following foods are likely to contain GMOs:

- Soy
- Corn
- Canola oil
- Sugar beets
- Cottonseed oil
- Dairy
- Papaya
- Zucchini
- Sugar (except cane sugar, which probably does not contain GMOs)
- Atlantic Salmon (approved November 2015)

The majority of processed foods contain some form of corn and soy. Cottonseed and canola oils are also used in a variety of packaged foods. One way to avoid GMOs is to eat organic foods and look for "non-GMO" on the label.

6) Read Food Labels. If the food you are purchasing has a label, know how to read the ingredient list. Remember that the front of the packaging is meant to sell, not to inform. The back of the package is where you'll find useful information. Many people just look at the grams of carbohydrates, fat, and protein, which don't tell you anything about the quality of the ingredients. It's more important to read the actual ingredients.

- Choose foods with few ingredients. Less than five, you get an A.

- The ingredient list should be recognizable and sound like a recipe, not a science experiment.

- Avoid foods that have more than 10 grams of sugar per serving. Most processed foods are high in sugar, even non-sweet foods like ketchup and salad dressings. Hidden sugars include maltodextrin, corn sweetener, barley malt, corn syrup, fruit juice concentrate, and ingredients ending in "–ose" or "–ol."

- Avoid foods containing high fructose corn syrup.

- Avoid anything "partially hydrogenated" or "hydrogenated." These are trans-fats: chemically altered fats that do not occur in nature.

- Avoid "white foods" made of processed flour, including most breads, crackers, chips, and pasta. Processed flour is quickly broken down into sugar, which elevates your blood sugar and promotes inflammation. Look for the word "whole" in front of the grain, which indicates it is less processed. More on this topic in Food Myths, below.

- Avoid artificial colors and flavors.

- Avoid MSG (monosodium glutamate) or anything "autolyzed" or "hydrolyzed," which probably contains MSG. This neurological stimulant can cause symptoms such as hyperactivity, headaches, palpitations, chest pain, and weakness.

- Avoid nitrates (sodium nitrite) used in processed meats, which are linked to heart disease, diabetes, and cancer. Most stores offer non-nitrate lunch meats, salami, and bacon, but these should still be eaten sparingly.

- Avoid artificial sweeteners. Many recent studies have shown that artificial sweeteners raise your blood sugar more than sugar,[42] cause obesity, and destroy the gut microbiome.

- And finally, eat more whole foods—those that don't have a food label but are already in their natural state (see next page).

7) Regain Control of What You Eat. Learn to cook, or at least purchase whole foods and prepare them at home. We are all capable of cutting up fruits and vegetables, boiling eggs, dividing nuts into portions, and assembling meals such as "Salad in a Jar" or "Overnight Oatmeal" (see the basic recipes in Chapter 14).

On any given day, 57% of Americans and a whopping 70% of teens are eating out at a restaurant instead of at home.[43] When you eat out, you give up control of your food quality, but that doesn't mean you can't eat out. Find restaurants that offer options for organic produce, grass-fed beef, free-range organic poultry, sustainable seafood, and locally sourced foods. More and more restaurants are taking this approach because of consumer demand. Food activists like Vani Hari (aka "The Food Babe") are campaigning effectively for change in quality, demanding that food companies and restaurant chains become transparent about food ingredients and remove potentially harmful chemicals from their food. This clean food movement has been gaining momentum, putting pressure on food companies to provide what people want—clean and healthier food choices.

8) Just Eat Real, Clean Food.

- Colorful fresh vegetables such as kale, spinach, broccoli, artichokes, avocados, asparagus, carrots, pumpkins, and onions, and colorful fruits such as blueberries, cranberries, blackberries, raspberries, strawberries, apples, and cherries.

- Legumes such as kidney beans, black beans, garbanzo beans, pinto beans, black-eyed peas, adzuki, and lima beans. If you buy canned beans, make sure the cans are BPA free to reduce exposure to this dangerous chemical.

- Clean and sustainable seafood such as wild salmon, mackerel, anchovies, sardines, bay scallops, clams, and mussels. (Refer to the EDF Seafood Selector.)

- Organic, free-range poultry/pork and grass-fed beef that has been raised humanely.

- Whole grains such as quinoa, millet, barley, oatmeal, cracked or sprouted wheat, and wild rice. If you have unexplained health problems, talk to your doctor about testing for celiac and gluten intolerance to see if you should avoid gluten-containing grains.

- Nuts and seeds such as walnuts, pecans, almonds, Brazil nuts, sunflower seeds, sesame seeds, and pumpkin seeds. Nuts and seeds are rich in minerals, trace elements, and healthy fats.

- Olive and coconut oil and grass-fed butter or ghee. Do not eat highly processed oils, such as canola or "vegetable" oils, or fried foods that contain trans-fats. For high heat cooking, use light olive oil, avocado oil, or high oleic sunflower oil.

- Grass-fed, organic dairy including plain, full-fat organic yogurt and small amounts of soft or aged cheese such as feta, goat cheese, or parmesan.

- Coconut, rice, or almond milk. These are good substitutes for cow's milk, which can cause sensitivities and inflammation.

- Fermented foods such as yogurt, kefir, kombucha, kimchi, sauerkraut, and other pickled vegetables. These contain good bacteria and support the microbiome.

- Fresh herbs and spices, which are loaded with antioxidants.

- Water, green tea, and organic coffee.

- Sweeteners in moderation, such as raw honey, real maple syrup, or raw cane or coconut sugar.

- Dark chocolate, sorbet, or gelato.

The Most Important Change You Should Make

If you could only make one change in your diet that would reduce your risk of premature death by 42 percent, your risk of cancer by 25 percent, and your risk of heart disease by 31 percent,[44] would you make that change? It is simple: Eat more plants.

In July 2014, a remarkable study was published by Dr. Esselstyn and colleagues in the *American Journal of Family Practice*. They recruited 198 people who had coronary artery disease. Many of these patients had been told they were not surgical candidates and that there was no other treatment option. Dr. Esselstyn put them on a very unconventional treatment—a vegan diet with no added oils and limited sugars and processed grains.

Eighty-nine percent of the patients were able to follow what many people would consider a "drastically limited" diet. Researchers found that an impressive 81 percent of the patients following the diet had improvement in their symptoms and 99 percent avoided any further cardiac event. [45] This is compared to 62 percent worsening in the patients who did not follow the diet.

Sadly, this study got little press. Once again, if a drug showed this kind of promise, every doctor in the country would know about it.

Plants contain phytonutrients, a plant component that provides their medicinal qualities. *"Phyto"* in Greek means "plants" and phytonutrients fall into their own nutrient category because they are not related to fats, carbohydrates, proteins, vitamins, or minerals. Phytonutrients add crucial information for your body, optimizing cellular function and communication. Many of these important components also act as antioxidants, neutralizing free radicals (unstable molecules that can promote inflammation and damage to the body tissues). In addition, phytonutrients have been shown to affect genes that control the growth of cancer cells (see below).

Plant foods are by far the most important component of our diet, promoting health and fighting disease. Plant fiber supports important detoxification components, healthy bowel movements, and a healthy microbiome. Certain fibers in vegetables contain prebiotics, which is food for the good bacteria. I recommend eating at least seven servings of veggies, primarily using the ratio of five servings of veggies and two of fruits, as fruits do contain more sugar. A good rule of thumb is that half of your plate at each meal should be made up of vegetables.

Cancer-Fighting Foods

Cancer is a multifactorial disease, a "perfect storm" so to speak, because genetic, environmental, and lifestyle factors can influence the development of cancer. We can control many of our environmental and lifestyle factors, especially what we eat. Certain plant foods have been shown to protect against cancer. So how does something as simple as eating vegetables prevent cancer? Plant foods fight disease in many ways.

Plant fiber assists the gut in eliminating waste, since plants contain nutrients that help the liver detoxify more efficiently. Certain plant nutrients have also been shown to switch on the genes that fight cancer and switch off the genes that allow cancer cells to grow out of control. Additionally, these important nutrients help improve function of the immune cells that fight cancer. There are thousands of studies supporting the role of plants in fighting cancer.[46]

The following is a summary of foods shown to have cancer-fighting properties and the primary component of the food thought to instill this beneficial effect.

- Garlic, onions, and leeks have immune-enhancing allium compounds that appear to increase the activity of the immune cells that fight cancer and indirectly help break down cancer-causing substances.[47]

- Cruciferous vegetables (broccoli, Brussels sprouts, cabbage, cauliflower, collards, kale, kohlrabi, mustard greens, rutabaga, and turnips) contain indole-3-carbinol (I3C) that may have a role in preventing hormone-linked cancers like breast and prostate cancers. I3C inhibits cancer cell growth, blocks the effects of estrogens, and helps rid the body of toxins.[48, 49, 50] Another component of broccoli, sulforaphane, switches off cancer-initiating genes and also helps the body detoxify. Sulforaphane has been shown to protect against cancers of the prostate, breast, bladder, and skin.[51, 52]

- Green and black teas contain a certain type of antioxidant, polyphenols (epigallocatechin-3-gallate, or ECGC), which appears to prevent growth of cancer cells and, in some studies, shows reduced risks of cancers of the colon, breast, ovary, prostate, and lung.[53, 54, 55, 56, 57, 58] Green teas are best, followed by the more common black tea. Herbal teas do not show this benefit.

- Omega-3 fatty acids from fatty fish and seeds like flax and chia have powerful anti-inflammatory effects and have evidence to support use in a variety of diseases associated with inflammation. It is likely that these anti-inflammatory effects are the reason why omega-3 fatty acids may be beneficial in cancer prevention, specifically colon, kidney, and breast cancers.[59, 60, 61]

Many supplement companies have isolated the above plant components and put them into capsules, promoting them for the prevention and treatment of cancers. Although it sounds good in theory, many studies show that eating foods rich in these components has a positive effect, but taking the isolated ingredient often does not confer the same benefit. It is very likely that these foods contain a variety of nutrients that work in conjunction to provide that anti-cancer effect.

Dispelling Common Food Myths

Myth: A calorie is a calorie.

I don't think anyone in the world would argue against the fact that you would be healthier if you ate 1,500 calories per day of fresh broccoli than if you ate 1,500 calories of hamburgers and fries. But that doesn't stop the food industry from creating products that are "low-calorie" or "low sugar," or claiming they are improving their products by making them lower in calories (which often just means changing the serving size). It doesn't stop us from using calorie-counting apps on our smartphones. It doesn't stop us from turning the package around to check the label for calorie content.

Although one calorie of any food has the same amount of energy from a chemistry standpoint, the way in which your body processes that calorie is much more complex. As I mentioned earlier, certain foods, such as sugar, stimulate the brain's addiction center. These foods have a major effect on the hormones that control hunger and your sense of fullness.

Remember that the foods you eat also feed your microbiome—the good bacteria that play a huge role in keeping you healthy. The rich combination of nutrients in whole foods regulates all of your metabolic processes, helps with detoxification, and decreases inflammation. Even more fascinating is that foods are information for your genes, as I described above.

Obviously, all calories are not created equal. To support your health, focus on eating calories that provide fuel and nutrition. Look at food as fuel and the building blocks to build a strong foundation leading to long-lasting health.

Myth: Whole wheat bread is better than white bread.

If I got a dollar for every time a patient told me proudly that they choose wheat bread over white bread, I would be rich. This is probably the food myth most taken advantage of by the food industry to sell a product. The difference between white flour and whole wheat flour is that white flour has had the outer layer of fiber and nutrients stripped from it. You are left with the inside of the grain—the starch—which is very quickly digested into sugar, leading to a rapid spike in blood sugar levels. If you read the ingredient list, you will see the words "enriched flour" because they are required to supplement the flour with vitamins that were stripped away in the process of making it. Flour is also commonly bleached, a chemical process simply done to make it look more appealing.

Most commercial "wheat bread" is not much different than white bread, other than containing some whole wheat and, frequently, caramel color to make it look brown. Manufacturers in the United States can call their bread "whole wheat" if it contains as little as 51 percent whole grains.[62] Caramel color is a potentially harmful additive that has been linked to cancer in animal studies.

Most wheat bread has the same effect as white bread on our blood sugar and insulin levels, promoting insulin resistance that leads to obesity and diabetes. Bread made with 100 percent whole grain is digested slower and doesn't cause as much spike in insulin levels; however, it is ultimately still broken down into sugar. Whole grain products do contain more fiber because the fiber hasn't been stripped off.

Another problem with wheat, whether white or whole grain, is that some people are sensitive to gluten, a protein component of wheat. Testing for gluten sensitivity has not yet been perfected and testing for celiac disease only detects the most severe response to gluten. Many people have sensitivity without having celiac disease, presenting as fatigue, headaches, bloating, constipation, diarrhea, weight gain, and brain fog. The best way to determine if you are sensitive is to cut out gluten completely from your diet for four weeks, then eat it and see if you have any symptoms. See the Resource section for more books about this problem.

Food products made from any type of flour are ultimately digested into sugar. So although it doesn't taste sweet, your body doesn't recognize the difference between digested flour and sugar. I often have patients keep a food diary and I show them how many equivalents of sugar they are actually consuming. You can do the same by calculating your net grams of carbohydrates using the following formula: Four grams of carbohydrates equals one teaspoon of sugar (excluding the fiber). For example, a medium bagel has 46 grams of carbohydrates and 2 grams of fiber, which is equivalent to 44 net grams (46 carbs minus 2 grams of fiber), which is the equivalent of 11 teaspoons (44 divided by 4) of sugar when digested.

To illustrate this concept, I asked one patient about her diet and she told me that she "eats really healthy." Most doctors would quit asking questions about diet at that point, but I asked her to walk me through a typical day and tell me what she eats. This is what she said:

Breakfast: Yoplait yogurt, banana, and coffee with Splenda.

Lunch: Turkey sandwich on whole wheat bread with lettuce and a tomato slice, pretzels, and a bottle of "vitamin water."

Snack: Kashi protein bar and Starbucks Skinny Latte.

Dinner: Grilled chicken, whole wheat pasta, and salad with honey mustard dressing.

Snack: Weight Watchers Greek frozen yogurt bar.

This "healthy" diet doesn't sound so bad—until you count up the net carbs and discover she was eating 230 grams of carbs, which equates to 57 teaspoons of sugar! And she was eating only two servings of vegetables/fruits.

Now look at the healthier alternative:

Breakfast: Plain yogurt with ¼ cup blueberries, a teaspoon of honey, and 1 tablespoon chopped walnuts. Coffee with a teaspoon of raw sugar.

Lunch: Slice of toasted Ezekiel sprouted bread with ½ avocado, tomato slices, and fresh ground pepper and sea salt, carrot wedges, and a club soda with fresh lime.

Snack: 15 gluten-free crackers with 1 tablespoon almond butter and a small apple.

Dinner: Grilled chicken, sweet potato, and broccoli.

Snack: 2 squares dark chocolate.

I would argue that this isn't an enormous change. And if you don't like anything above, there are plenty of substitutes that would still be low in processed carbohydrates and sugar. This daily menu contains 92 grams of carbohydrates, equating to 23 teaspoons of sugar. With those small changes, she cut her carbohydrate intake in half and doubled her intake of fruits and veggies.

Carbohydrates, as a whole nutrient category, are not inherently bad for you. It is the quality of carbohydrates that is important. Carbohydrates that are naturally present in plant foods like veggies, fruits, nuts, beans, and whole grains are wonderful sources of vitamins, minerals, phytonutrients, and fiber. These can also be considered "slow carbs"— ones that are digested slowly and contain fiber that helps your gut function optimally.

"Bad carbs," or "fast carbs," come from sugar and processed grains stripped of their fiber component. In addition, the quantity of carbohydrates in the standard American diet—as described in the former example above—is just too much energy in the form of sugar than most of us need in a day.

Myth: Fat is your enemy.

For decades, fat has been vilified by the media. One of the biggest health misconceptions is that fats, as a whole category, need to be avoided in order to lose weight, prevent heart disease, control diabetes, and lower cholesterol. The truth is that healthy fats, especially monounsaturated fats and essential fatty acids (omegas 3 & 6), are essential to your health, especially your blood vessels, heart, and brain.

Many studies dispelling the myth of the low-fat diet have been published in respected journals such as the *American Journal of Clinical Nutrition*,[63, 64, 65, 66] *New England Journal of Medicine*,[67, 68, 69] *Journal of Clinical Endocrinology*,[70, 71] *Diabetic Medicine*,[72, 73] *Journal of Pediatrics*,[74, 75] and *Nutrition and Metabolism*.[76, 77] These studies, comparing low-fat/high carbohydrate diets to high-fat/lower carbohydrate diets, have repeatedly demonstrated that higher fat diets had the greatest improvement in weight loss, blood pressure, blood sugar, triglycerides, cholesterol, and cognitive function.[78, 79, 80, 81, 82, 83, 84, 85]

With regard to fat intake and cancer risk, this is even a more complex area. For years, scientists and researchers thought that a high intake of dietary fat increased the risk of breast and prostate cancer. However, it is more likely that the risk of hormone-dependent cancers have more to do with obesity than fat intake. Fat cells store estrogen and also create inflammation, the combination that promotes growth of these cancers.[86] Another factor is probably the deleterious effect of the unhealthy fat sources Americans eat, as discussed earlier.

Since the 1970s, when low-fat diets began to be recommended by "experts" and there was an explosion of low-fat and non-fat foods in the market, the rate of increase in diabetes and obesity more than doubled. Studies show that an intake of monounsaturated fats, like olive oil, is associated with a decreased risk of high blood pressure, heart attack, diabetes, "bad" LDL cholesterol, cancer, and inflammation.[87,88,89,90,91] Healthy monounsaturated and omega-3 fats come from nuts, seeds, avocados, and (wild) fatty fish.

The types of fat you eat are much more important than the total intake. For example, a study comparing corn oil to olive oil showed that corn oil switches off the genes that suppress breast cancer, where olive oil does not have the same effect.[92] We need to get away from the notion of lumping all fats, carbohydrates, and proteins together and pay much more attention to the nutritional quality and type of fat, carbohydrates, or protein.

As previously discussed, the worst fats are chemically altered, trans-fats added to packaged and processed foods to increase shelf life and thus increase profits for food manufacturers. Stop eating foods that come in a box or a bag. And please stop eating fake butter—99 percent of the butter substitutes contain hydrogenated fats! To quote a mentor and Functional Medicine neurologist, Dr. Perlmutter, "I can't believe it's not butter? I can't believe people eat this stuff."[93]

Keep in mind that the food companies can label a food as having "no trans-fats" if it contains less than ½ gram of trans-fats per serving, so always look for trans-fats in the ingredient list. Do not eat foods containing "partially hydrogenated" or "hydrogenated" oils—these are trans-fats.

Avoid highly processed oils, especially generic "vegetable oils," soybean oil, and canola oil. Most vegetable oils are made from GMOs and are highly processed—extracted with toxic solvents, refined, bleached, and deodorized to make them colorless, odorless, and tasteless, retaining only their calories. The extensive processing removes any nutritional value the original plant may have contained.

Instead look for expeller-pressed oils such as extra virgin olive oil, grape seed oil, walnut oil, avocado oil, sesame oil, or coconut oil. Good old-fashioned butter (from grass-fed cows producing organic milk) is also a great option. Some oils are not stable at high temperatures and should not be used for high heat cooking. Ideas on how to buy, use, and store cooking oils can be found in the Resource section.

Myth: Eggs are bad for you.

A review of food myths would not be complete if we didn't address the vilification of the egg. Eggs are quite possibly one of the most perfect protein sources on this earth. The main reason that eggs have been vilified is the cholesterol content of the yolk. You will learn in the next section that it has finally been determined that dietary cholesterol is not behind the epidemic of heart disease.

But be sure you are eating eggs from chickens raised in a healthy and humane way, rather than eggs from unhealthy chickens. A 2010 study from Penn State University showed that hens that were kept outside in pastures, rather than in a cage, laid eggs that contained twice as much vitamin E and 2½ times the amount of omega-3 fatty acids than the eggs from their cooped-up counterparts.[94]

Eggs are one of the healthiest and most affordable sources of protein. Essential to the health of the eye and maintenance of good vision, egg yolks contain lutein and zeaxanthin that prevent macular degeneration and cataracts. Supplements containing lutein and zeaxanthin are prescribed by ophthalmologists, but these nutrients are much better absorbed when they are obtained from the diet along with all the other beneficial nutrients, and the egg yolk is a perfect source. Studies show that just one egg per day increases these two important nutrients and also results in an increase of the protective pigment in the eye.[95, 96]

So don't throw away the yolk! The majority of the nutrients and half of the protein are contained in it. A study at the University of Connecticut found that the fat in egg yolks actually helps to reduce your bad cholesterol and improve blood sugar.[97] Throwing away the yolk is throwing away the best part: essential omega-3 fats, B vitamins, calcium, and vitamins A and D. Trust Mother Nature—all those ingredients are there for a reason.

Contrary to popular belief, eggs do not increase your risk of heart disease, and they actually may reduce the incidence of stroke by preventing clotting and inflammation.[98] Eggs also contain choline, which is important for the health of our cells, especially in the brain and nervous system.

Do not eat store-bought egg whites in a carton! These products take advantage of the myth that the fat and cholesterol in the yolk are bad for your health. They remove the yolks and then add synthetic vitamins, additives, and preservatives. And why do they add all those synthetic vitamins to the egg whites? Because they removed the vitamins when they removed the yolk!

You may recall from previous chapters that eggs are on the list of trigger foods that can cause sensitivity or inflammation in the gut. If you think you might have poor gut health or food sensitivities, following the four-week elimination diet described in Chapter 4 can help you determine if you have sensitivity to eggs. If you don't, then they are a very healthy addition to your diet.

Myth: Cholesterol causes heart disease.

Cholesterol is an essential structural component of every cell in your body. Twenty-five percent of that cholesterol is found in your brain and is critical to the function of chemical messengers, as well as the outer lining of nerve cells in your brain.[99] Cholesterol is also the building block for important hormones like estrogen, testosterone, progesterone, and vitamin D. In addition, it is important for the digestion of fats. Cholesterol is not an enemy contained in your food. Eighty percent of cholesterol is produced by your body because your body needs it. So why has cholesterol become the villain?

When autopsies in the early 1900s revealed that plaques in the coronary arteries contained lots of cholesterol, it was assumed that cholesterol was the culprit. For almost 50 years, the government has been telling us to remove cholesterol from our diet. The food industry answered by producing lots of cholesterol-free foods, but heart disease has continued to rise to epidemic proportions.

In 2015, the Dietary Guidelines Advisory Committee concluded that the evidence shows no appreciable relationship between consumption of dietary cholesterol and blood cholesterol. They deemed—after 50 years of drilling into us that cholesterol is the enemy—that "cholesterol is not a nutrient of concern."[100] We now know that it is an innocent bystander, NOT a villain. What happens to cholesterol in the presence of inflammation is the real problem.

Drug companies followed the opportunity made by cholesterol's critics and produced a class of medications called statins. These cholesterol-lowering medicines have become the top-selling drugs in America, with one in four Americans over the age of 45 taking a statin. Are these drugs benefiting us?

You have all heard about "good cholesterol" (HDL) and "bad cholesterol" (LDL). These are actually misnomers. LDL and HDL are not types of cholesterol, but carrier proteins (vehicles) that transport cholesterol (the passenger) around the body. A standard lipid panel (total cholesterol, LDL, HDL, and triglycerides) measures the amount of cholesterol carried by these "vehicles."

Although elevated LDL cholesterol is a risk factor for heart disease, there are now even more specific markers to determine the danger. The size of the vehicle contributes to the risk: the smaller and denser the "vehicle" (dense LDL), the higher the possibility that it can enter the wall of the blood vessel and form plaque. Oxidized LDL and Lp(a) are also subtypes of cholesterol and carrier proteins that indicate a higher heart disease risk. Testing subtypes of cholesterol and markers of inflammation, called advanced cholesterol testing, should be taken into consideration in assessing probability of heart disease, as well as tracking improvements in those levels. The more inflammation in the body, the more likely that plaque will become unstable, or break off and cause a heart attack or stroke.

Further discussion about the intricacies of cholesterol subtypes and cardiac risk markers is beyond the scope of this book. I will say that in my clinical practice, I do not hand out prescriptions for statins to everyone with elevated cholesterol. In fact, I do not recommend cholesterol-lowering medication until I have fully evaluated all risk factors: advanced cholesterol testing, inflammation markers, and a Coronary Artery Calcium score (CAC). A very good predictor of heart disease risk, the CAC test uses a low-radiation, limited CT scan to measure plaque in the coronary arteries. Multiple studies over the past ten years support using CAC scores for determining cardiac risk.[101,102,103,104,105] Furthermore, patients with a CAC score of zero are unlikely to benefit from cholesterol medications.[106]

A CAC score is a much better predictor than the esteemed Framingham score that most physicians are taught to rely on in order to determine their patient's cardiac risk.[107][108] In 2013, the Framingham rules were revised to a new scoring system. This new and improved scoring system, rather than using other tests to identify those patients that might not benefit from statins, would result in an estimated 20 million more statin prescriptions being written. Many of the panel members were affiliated with pharmaceutical companies, and the studies used to back the guidelines were funded by pharmaceutical companies.

Despite the strong evidence supporting the use of CAC scores, primary care physicians rarely order this test and most patients have never heard of it. I wonder if the fact that insurance does not yet cover it has any influence on its underutilization. How many patients are on unnecessary cholesterol medications because they have never had this test? If insurance doesn't cover it, then it must be costly, right? Wrong! The test costs under $200.

Patients with a lower risk, or no evidence of heart disease, should be shown how to improve their numbers with lifestyle changes such as nutrition, exercise, stress reduction, weight loss, and smoking cessation. Although most (if not all) physicians would probably agree this is the most effective way to improve cardiac risk markers, few doctors have the time or training to guide their patients. I have seen patients decrease their LDL by over 100 points simply by changing what they eat (and it was not a low-fat, low-cholesterol diet). I have seen similar results with exercise alone. Lifestyle is a much more powerful medicine than anything a drug company can produce.

So why should we be concerned about taking statin medications? Remember, cholesterol is an essential component of the body. We don't know the long-term effects of driving the total cholesterol numbers down very low. Statin medications also reduce levels of CoQ10, a vital substance produced by your body and used by every cell for energy production, cell growth, and muscle contraction. Statins can cause fatigue and muscle pain, probably due to the interference of your body's production of CoQ10. In some patients, statins can cause cognitive problems (poor memory, difficulty concentrating, and depression). These drugs also increase your risk of developing diabetes by up to 46 percent.[109]

Isn't it ironic that we are treating one risk factor for heart disease (high cholesterol) and at the same time increasing the risk of another condition (diabetes) that causes the very condition we're attempting to prevent?

I'm concerned that Americans are being over-treated with medications and not being provided with up-to-date advice on the role of nutrition, or how to adequately assess cardiac risk. Although statins have been shown to reduce the risk of heart attack in patients with heart disease, evidence to support their use in those without heart disease is weak. Furthermore, statin medications do not address the underlying problem of inflammation, which is most often caused by the everyday personal health choices being made.

Keep in mind that statins are a billion-dollar business for the pharmaceutical industry. The majority of studies are funded by this industry and, unfortunately, it is where doctors get their information— from those directly benefiting from the sale of the drugs. This is certainly a conflict of interest.

If you are taking a statin, do not stop taking it. Talk to your doctor about whether you need it given your individual situation, and don't be afraid to ask detailed questions. If you already have heart disease, it may be best to stay on the medication. If you don't have heart disease, ask for a coronary calcium score to see if you already have plaque in your coronary arteries.

Take control of your health and make the changes you need to improve it. If you want a more individualized approach, more comprehensive testing, and guidance on the right lifestyle changes, consider seeing a Functional Medicine physician (see Resources).

Valerie's Story

Valerie came to me with the simple goals of eating healthier, feeling better, and potentially getting off the statin medication she was put on for high cholesterol. After talking more with her about her current health, it was apparent she wasn't doing as well as she appeared.

She had a long history of migraine headaches that had increased in frequency over the past several years, to the point that she was having headaches about 2–4 times per month. She had fatigue, poor sleep, difficult concentrating, and muscle pain, and felt like she constantly had the flu. There were many days when she just couldn't function at all. Constipation and bloating had plagued her for as long as she could remember.

Valerie was so accustomed to feeling bad that she didn't remember what it was like to feel good. Her prescription drug regimen included daily medications for sleep and migraine prevention, along with the statin to lower her cholesterol that she had been taking for several years. When she went to see her doctor complaining of the above symptoms, she was told she probably had fibromyalgia and Chronic Fatigue Syndrome. More medications were recommended. She decided the answers she was getting from conventional medicine were not acceptable, so she came to me for an alternative approach.

After discontinuing the statin and removing gluten from her diet, her sleep improved, her muscle pain resolved, she had better energy, and she started to lose weight. She then cut out dairy and the constipation she had for years also resolved. Through a lot of experimentation with food and listening to her body, she discovered that a clean, Paleo-type diet suited her. Making those changes gave her more strength, better sleep, and more energy.

And what happened with her high cholesterol? Initially after she went off the statin, her LDL (bad cholesterol) went up to 146 (the optimal level is less than 100). But after making the dietary changes described above and adding some nutritional supplements, Valerie's LDL dropped to 76...without medication. She was also able to reduce her Lp(a), the high-risk cholesterol subtype, by half. Her blood sugar levels, which were initially in the borderline pre-diabetic range, dropped to an optimal level.

Most importantly, the way she feels now is completely different, "like night and day." Instead of feeling foggy, tired, and achy, she feels awake, present, and healthy, and is 20 pounds lighter. She feels healthier than she has in years.

There are several learning points from Valerie's story. Symptoms from gluten and other food sensitivities are often very subtle and can present with non-specific signs, such as migraines, fatigue, poor sleep, and chronic constipation. Conventional medicine's knee-jerk reaction is almost always medication; however, there is nothing more powerful than food.

If the cause of her symptoms had been recognized early on, she would have never needed the migraine and sleep medication. And if she had been treated with nutritional changes initially, Valerie would have likely never been recommended to be put on a statin, which caused her fatigue to worsen, as well as caused muscle weakness and difficulty exercising. Both the statin and gluten were likely behind her difficulty losing weight.

This case is a great example of the quote at the beginning of the chapter: food can be the slowest form of poison or the most powerful medicine. In Valerie's case, she experienced both and emerged as a new person.

A Few Words about Supplements

A thorough discussion of supplements is beyond the scope of this book and could be a book of its own. I will say that it is always best to get your nutrients from foods. Whole, plant foods are packaged by nature in a way that the whole is greater than the sum of its parts.

With that being said, the majority of people do not eat adequate amounts of plant foods. Furthermore, the nutrient content of crops has declined over the years. A landmark study, published in 2004, demonstrated that nutrient content has declined as much as 38% since the 1950's.[110] For these reasons, I do take supplements and prescribe them to my patients. When necessary, I also prescribe other specific vitamins, minerals, nutrients, and herbs for certain medical conditions.

The following are my general recommendations regarding supplements:

- Supplements are meant to complement your diet and provide what you might be missing. Always strive to get your nutrients from a healthy diet.
- For most patients, I recommend a multivitamin/multimineral, omega-3, vitamin D and probiotic.
- It is very important to take high-quality supplements that are tested by a third party to ensure they contain the stated ingredients, contain the most bioavailable and best absorbed forms of the nutrients, and do not contain unnecessary

additives and preservatives. Most over-the-counter brands are not good quality. A good giveaway is that quality supplements don't offer BOGO (buy one, get one free) deals!

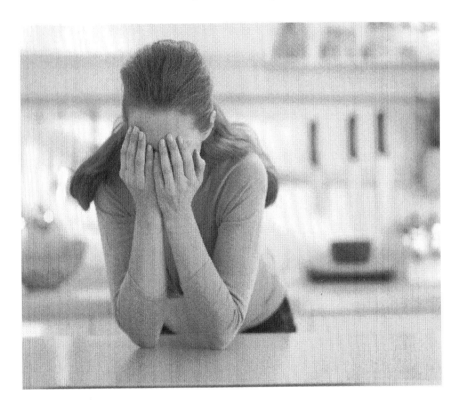

CHAPTER SEVEN

STEP FOUR: KEEP STRESS FROM KILLING YOU

It's not stress that kills us, it is our reaction to it.
~ Hans Selye

Stress and Disease

We all know that stress is bad for our health. It is linked to all chronic disease—diabetes, obesity, high blood pressure, heart disease, gastrointestinal problems like irritable bowel and acid reflux, depression and anxiety, allergies and asthma, autoimmune disease, fibromyalgia, and more.

Once you are aware of the physiologic basis of the stress response, you will see clearly why stress has these deleterious effects on the body. And when you understand why stress is a slow, silent killer, you can appreciate the power of stress reduction in improving your health.

Stress is a good thing when it comes to short-term problems. The fight-or-flight response is the body's reaction that allows us to escape from something bad. What happens inside your body that prepares you for the fight-or-flight response?

- Your heart rate goes up.
- Your blood pressure increases.
- Blood sugar increases to give you energy.
- Your muscles tense up, ready for action.
- Blood flow to your gut decreases.
- You become more mentally alert.
- Your immune system is suppressed.

Acute stress is a good thing because it helps your body adapt to a threat. It allows you to be faster and stronger in order to fight the enemy. It redirects your body's resources away from digestion and immunity, since you don't need those functions when you are in danger. It puts you on high alert mentally so you can be aware of the threat.

With chronic stress, these effects are not good because all those responses happen constantly at a lower level. The physiologic effects that are supposed to help you eventually begin to hurt you:

- The increase in blood pressure becomes hypertension.
- The elevated blood sugar becomes diabetes.
- Your muscle tension becomes chronic tension-type headache, or neck and back pain.
- The decreased blood flow to the gut results in heartburn, upset stomach, diarrhea, or constipation.
- Your constant mental alertness becomes chronic anxiety.
- Decreased immunity makes you more susceptible to infection.

Chronic elevation of the stress hormone, cortisol, also makes you gain weight. Cortisol causes your body to crave high-calorie foods, like fats and carbohydrates, and to store fat around your organs. This highly inflammatory visceral fat, also known as belly fat, not only gives you a "muffin top" or "beer belly," but also increases your risk of chronic disease.

Elevated cortisol disrupts hormone balance on all fronts, wreaking havoc on the body in so many ways. It increases insulin resistance—causing your cells to be less responsive to insulin—thus increasing risk of diabetes. Elevated cortisol disrupts production of your reproductive hormones, contributing to low testosterone in men and women, changes in menstrual periods, and worsening of menopausal symptoms.

High levels of cortisol can also make your thyroid dysfunctional in a multitude of ways. It disrupts every facet of the thyroid cascade, from the brain to the thyroid gland to how well your cells respond to thyroid hormone. As mentioned in Chapter 3, chronic stress can also increase the permeability of the gut. This may be why stress and trauma often precedes development of autoimmune disease.

Kathy's Story

Over and over again, I hear patients tell similar stories of how autoimmune disease presents—often with a trauma or very high-stress time immediately preceding the onset of flagrant symptoms. Stress causes severe imbalance in our bodies and often is the "final straw" in triggering the explosion of a smoldering problem.

In 2006, Kathy was a 42-year-old lieutenant colonel in the US Army on active duty in Iraq. As a combat commander, she was always under heightened alert and constantly under enemy fire. She had been sent back to combat repeatedly after suffering injuries from explosives. It was not only the physical injuries Kathy was experiencing, but emotional as well, after losing five of her close comrades. Stress was high, diet was poor, sleep was rare, and she was sustaining herself on Red Bull.

At the end of her mission, she had a sudden onset of back pain, leg weakness, and loss of vision. These symptoms resolved themselves initially, but over the next two years, she developed progressive fatigue, memory loss, visual changes, and leg spasms. Kathy was evaluated by many physicians and diagnosed with post-traumatic stress syndrome (PTSD). She was put on one medication after another for her symptoms—ironically some to treat the side effects of the other medications. By 2008, she was confined to a wheelchair, had severe depression, was taking 18 prescriptions, and felt like she was "in a fog."

After continuing to have progressive symptoms and ultimately losing her vision permanently, Kathy was evaluated at a large teaching hospital and finally diagnosed with MS in 2011. The next steps included powerful immune-suppressing MS drugs in addition to a cocktail of other medications for relief of symptoms. By 2011, she had hit rock bottom and attempted suicide by overdose. Fortunately, she wasn't successful.

The one thing in Kathy's life motivating her to pull herself out of what seemed like a hopeless situation was that she desperately wanted to see her grandchildren grow up. So after five years of frustrating doctor visits and a litany of powerful drugs with horrible side effects, she decided to try something drastic.

In 2012, she stopped most of the prescription drugs and focused on improving her lifestyle. Kathy cut alcohol, sugar, and processed foods from her diet and very slowly started getting back to moving her body. One day at a time, she began to feel better. She practiced yoga and relaxation exercises to help with her anxiety. Kathy's guide dog, George, was another source of emotional support. In 2013, she had recovered enough that she was able to start training for triathlons, and subsequently completed the St. Anthony's triathlon in St. Petersburg, Florida.

When she came to see me in late 2013, she was still struggling with poor sleep, anxiety and PTSD, joint pain, hot flashes, mood swings, and fatigue, which Kathy thought was the best she could expect given her medical condition. She was taking oral estrogen for hormone replacement and medications for sleep, depression, and panic attacks. Her blood work showed signs of inflammation, with hsCRP levels very high at 6.0 (normal is less than 1.0), her "bad cholesterol" (LDL) was 160 (optimal is less than 100), and a high-risk cardiac marker, Lp(a), was elevated at 62 (normal is less than 30). Her vitamin D and omega-3 levels were extremely low.

The approach for Kathy was simple—clean up her diet even more, correct her vitamin D deficiency, supplement with high-dose fish oil to decrease inflammation, and balance her hormones more effectively with bioidentical hormone pellets (see next chapter).

After one year, her hsCRP had decreased to normal (0.8), her LDL was down to 117, and her Lp(a) had decreased by 50 percent. She was off all medications, the majority of her symptoms had resolved, and she was sleeping better than she had in decades. In addition, she became more lean, with a ten-pound shift in body composition (a ten-pound fat loss offset by a ten-pound muscle gain). Kathy's energy and strength are more than she could have imagined. She was selected for the US Paralympic cycling team, moving up to second ranking and beating out competitors half her age.

Most importantly, she recently went to the beach with her grandsons and was frolicking, chasing, wrestling, and hiking with them, something she had only dreamed about doing five years ago. Rather than being disabled and living "in a fog," she is now living a meaningful, active life. Wanting to give back to those who are suffering, Kathy is starting a non-profit called True North, helping to heal wounded soldiers and civilians who are suffering from similar trauma, injuries, and disease with a holistic, natural approach.

Kathy's amazing story of recovery required a belief that she could find another solution to her condition. It took years of commitment and persistence in believing in the process and making small, daily changes that altered her destination forever.

Ways to Reduce Cortisol Levels

The most powerful way to reduce stress is through your body's natural relaxation mechanisms. Reducing cortisol levels takes a little time on your part, but it is well worth it. There is a powerful connection between the mind and the body.

So how do you lower cortisol levels? There are many different approaches—yet all are simple. The following activities reduce your cortisol by the following percentages:

- Listening to relaxing music—66 percent.[111]
- Increasing your sleep from six to eight hours—50 to 80 percent.[112]
- A good laugh—47 percent.[113]
- Getting a massage—31 percent.[114]
- Cutting out caffeine—30 percent.[115]
- Practicing meditation—20 percent.[116]

The Power of Breath

The stress response is regulated by a part of your nervous system called the "autonomic nervous system" (ANS). You don't have to think about breathing or direct your gut to digest your food or remind your heart to pump. The ANS keeps everything going on in the background, like your computer's operating system. There is, however, one autonomic function we do have control over—our breath.

You can hold your breath, change your breathing pattern, or decide to take deep breaths or shallow breaths, and it is the one and only direct link to the ANS. Breathing can control heart rate, blood pressure, gut function, and muscle tension—all of the physiologic changes that happen when the fight-or-flight stress response occurs. As the bridge to your ANS, breathing is a very powerful tool in reducing stress, and thus your risk of chronic disease.

I often demonstrate this with patients. For example, I had a patient who came into the office with a blood pressure of 180/90. I knew she had a lot of stress in her life, so I said, "I want to show you something." I had her lie down in the exam room and guided her through a controlled breathing exercise (listed below). I told her to repeat the exercise for the next five minutes and left the room.

When I returned, I rechecked her blood pressure and it was 150/80. That is the power of breath! Typical blood pressure medication cannot cause such an immediate reduction—never mind with no cost and no side effects.

Practice Deep Breathing: The 4-7-8 Exercise

- Exhale completely through your mouth.
- Close your mouth and inhale slowly and steadily through your nose while you silently count to four.
- Hold your breath while you silently count to seven.
- Exhale completely through your mouth, counting to eight.
- Repeat the process three times.

The Power of Sleep

Stress and sleep are closely intertwined. When we are stressed, we sleep less. Conversely, when we don't get enough sleep, we are less able to handle stress. Lack of sleep has an enormous impact on our health, particularly increasing risk of chronic disease.

Let me give you an analogy about sleep. When you go to Disney World, you notice it is sparkling clean, there is beautiful landscaping, and the rides rarely break down. The staff constantly keeps the place looking like the "happiest place on earth." But what would happen if Disney World never closed? When they close the park, they clean it, maintain the rides, take care of the gardening, and make everything look beautiful.

What would happen if you never closed? Sleep is the time when your body "cleans house," does most of its repair work, and regenerates your body's structure. Human growth hormone (HGH), also known as the "fountain of youth" hormone, is released during the sleep cycle to direct the repairs. Other hormones released during sleep help regulate your appetite, which is why poor sleep increases the risk of obesity. Sleep is also vital to a healthy immune system—so you get sick easier when you are sleep deprived.

Most importantly, during sleep is when your DNA is repaired. DNA damage leads to cancer and accelerated aging. There is no shortage of studies demonstrating the link between inadequate sleep and cancer— increased risk of breast, colon, and prostate cancer, promotion of tumor growth, and increased risk of cancer progression.[117,118,119,120] The probable connection is that inadequate sleep increases inflammation and also causes an imbalance of hormones, promoting cancer growth.[121]

Many studies demonstrate that sleep deprivation can cause a wide range of other disorders and issues, including obesity, high blood pressure, diabetes, heart disease, and more. Sleeping less than five hours a night increases your risk for heart attack by 48 percent and stroke by 15 percent.[122] Another study demonstrated that consistently sleeping less than five hours per night increased the risk of premature death—from all causes—by 15 percent.[123]

Excess sleep is not good either, with some increased risk of disease from sleeping over eight hours. It appears that the sweet spot is seven to eight hours, but we're all different. You have to judge whether you feel rested when you wake up or not. Infants and children require more sleep than adults, from 8–14 hours depending on the age. Babies need the most sleep, but this need declines as you progress toward adulthood.

Nine Steps to Restful Sleep

The most effective way to improve your sleep is to change your habits around sleep. Healthy sleep habits promote a normal circadian rhythm, which is the part of your brain that signals when it is time to sleep and when it is time to wake up.

1) Make a bedtime schedule. To set your internal clock, get up and go to bed as close to the same time as possible every day.

2) Create a relaxing bedtime routine. A soothing or relaxing activity at least 30 to 60 minutes before bed, such as reading, listening to music, or taking a bath is essential to prepare your body for sleep. You can also add Epsom salts (that contain magnesium) and essential oils, such as lavender, to your bath, both of which promote relaxation. Make it a point to not use any digital devices, such as your phone, laptop, or TV, for an hour before bed because these stimulate wakefulness. This is the hard part for most of us!

3) Avoid caffeine in the afternoon or evening. Caffeine, not surprisingly, can interfere with sleep, so avoid drinking anything caffeinated for 6–8 hours before bedtime.

4) Regular exercise promotes good sleep. However, exercising too close to bedtime may interfere with sleep. It is best to exercise first thing in the morning to improve mood and energy throughout the day.

5) Have a small, healthy snack before going to bed. A good bedtime snack is a few walnuts and a cup of decaffeinated herbal tea (chamomile or lavender). Walnuts help boost your melatonin level, the sleep hormone that controls your sleep cycle.

6) Keep your room as dark as possible while sleeping. Eliminate any electronics that emit blue light, as it can disrupt sleep.

7) Expose yourself to natural sunlight as soon after waking as possible. This signals your brain that it is time to be awake. It is very important to use your body's own circadian signals to keep your sleep cycle regular.

8) Keep your room cool. A room temperature of 65–72° Fahrenheit can enhance your quality of sleep.

9) Use your bed only for sleep and sex. If you wake up and can't go back to sleep, get up and do something else. Don't watch TV or use the computer or other electronics while in bed.

The Power of Positivity

Many studies show that a positive attitude is associated with better health: better immune system function, better heart health, more energy, and better sleep quality.

Heart Health

Researchers at Duke University Medical Center tracked the psychological and physical health of more than 2,800 patients diagnosed with heart disease. They found the patients who were initially optimistic about their treatment and recovery were more likely to be alive after 15 years than patients with similar diseases who had a more negative attitude.[124] A Johns Hopkins study demonstrated that a positive attitude was associated with nearly a 50 percent reduction in heart disease in the highest risk patients.[125]

Anti-Aging

Another study through University of Texas followed 1,550 initially healthy patients and found that those with a positive attitude were far less likely to show development of frailty and decline in function.[126] Researchers from Yale also found that those with a positive attitude live seven years longer than their "glass half empty" counterparts.[127]

Pain Reduction

A negative attitude also effects our perception of pain—a good example of the strong connection between the mind and the body. Studies show that people who have expectations of less pain experienced 30 percent less pain, which is as effective as a shot of morphine.[128]

There is no better example of the power of the mind than the use of hypnosis in pain management. Hypnosis has become common in the treatment of severe burns and has been shown to reduce pain intensity, improve effectiveness of pain medications, reduce anxiety, and improve wound healing.[129] There have even been many reports of people undergoing surgery with only the use of hypnosis.[130]

Four Ways to Improve Your Attitude

1) Be Grateful. It's impossible to be grateful and feel stressed at the same time. Try writing a gratitude list of everything you're happy for in your life. Every day when you wake up, or even just when you're stressed, take it out and read it.

2) Forgive Your Enemies. Anger and resentment toward others is an enormous source of stress. People who are prone to anger have a higher chance of heart disease—three times the risk, even in the absence of high blood pressure.[131]

Forgiveness doesn't mean that you forget, and it's not saying that what happened is okay. The decision to forgive is a gift that you give yourself.

It is also courageous and a sign of strength. As Mahatma Gandhi said, "The weak can never forgive. Forgiveness is an attribute of the strong."[132]

3) Let Go of What You Can't Control. I always like to think of the word "responsibility" being broken down into the words "response" and "ability"—meaning you have control of your response to the stressors, triggers, and people around you. There is a space between an event and your response that you have control over. You can pause and choose your response.

Taking responsibility for your reactions is a good tool for stress reduction. Another helpful idea that can reduce stress about circumstances that you can't control is to ask yourself, "Is this going to matter in five years?" If not, it's not worth stressing over.

4) Find Your Passion and Purpose. Choose to do something you enjoy every day for at least 30 minutes. Spending time on your passion and purpose decreases cortisol levels and the stress response. People who volunteer for an organization and who feel passionate about their work have better health outcomes.[133]

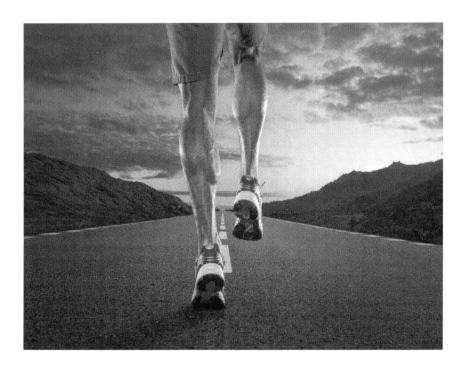

CHAPTER EIGHT

STEP FIVE: GET OUT OF YOUR CHAIR

What fits your schedule better, exercising 1 hour a day or being dead 24 hours per day?

~ Sonny Glasbergen, Cartoonist

The biggest bang for your buck in regards to promoting health and longevity is to get out of your chair. Alpa Patel, an epidemiologist at the American Cancer Society, tracked the health of 123,000 Americans between 1992 and 2006. The men in the study who spent more than six hours per day of their leisure time sitting had an overall death rate that was about 20 percent higher than the men who sat for three hours or less. And the death rate for women who sat for more than six hours a day was about 40 percent higher.[134] Unfortunately, movement is probably one of the least prescribed, proven treatments to prevent death and disease.

A Treatment for All Disease

Studies show that exercise, primarily light exercise such as 30 minutes of daily walking, has enormous benefits for disease prevention.[135, 136, 137, 138, 139] Exercise reduces these diseases and conditions by the following percentages:

- Diabetes—40–60 percent.
- Alzheimer's disease—50 percent.
- Anxiety and depression—48 percent.
- Arthritis pain—47 percent.
- Colon cancer—30–40 percent.
- Breast cancer—20–30 percent.
- Premature death from any cause—20–30 percent.

Studies show that exercise is as effective, if not more effective, than medications for the treatment of depression. But how often is it prescribed as a treatment of depression? How often do you think doctors say, "I can give you a prescription for Prozac or a prescription for exercise"?

Unfortunately, drug companies capitalize on our "pill for every ill" mindset. Ten percent of Americans take an anti-depressant medication, while only 20 percent of Americans meet the minimum recommendations for exercise.[140]

One remarkable study looked at the effect of exercise in 101 patients with coronary artery disease. Half of the patients were treated with surgery—having a stent placed in the blocked artery—and the other half were treated with exercise. After just one year, the surgery group was 70 percent free of recurrent chest pain or heart attack, and the exercise group was 88 percent free of disease. The exercise was more effective than surgery.[141]

Conventional medicine is quick to prescribe medication and surgery even when evidence shows that a lifestyle change, like adding or increasing exercise, can be more effective. Furthermore, exercise is much more cost effective—the average cost of surgery for heart disease is $30,000. Exercise is free.

Exercise Doesn't Take as Much Time as You Think

One of the biggest obstacles people seem to face with exercise is finding the time. We're all busy, and that's our favorite excuse. The optimal benefit of exercise appears to be about 30–60 minutes per day; however, any amount is better than none.[142]

Some evidence shows that a shorter workout at a higher intensity, known as High-Intensity Interval Training (HIIT) or "burst training," can be more effective than a longer workout. The benefits of interval training are that you burn more calories in a shorter period of time and increase your metabolism for 24–48 hours after your workout.

Interval training also helps you burn more fat and gain more muscle strength.[143, 144, 145] In the last chapter, I mentioned that HGH is known as the "fountain of youth" hormone, helping the body repair and regenerate. HIIT increases the release of HGH by 450 percent after an interval training session.[146] Injections of HGH are used as an anti-aging treatment and have been shown to increase lean body mass and decrease fat. Unfortunately, we don't know the long-term effects of using HGH. Some researchers are concerned it may stimulate growth of cancer cells. However, a HIIT workout that increases the body's own production of HGH has the benefits without the potential negative long-term effects.

HIIT has a significant potential for treatment of diabetes. We have long known that exercise lowers blood sugar levels. However, HIIT has the potential to rapidly reverse the insulin resistance that is at the root of the diabetes epidemic. HIIT starts reversing insulin resistance only 2 weeks after starting a HIIT exercise program.[147] We will discuss insulin resistance more in Chapter 10.

Tips for Interval Training & Exercising

Interval training simply alternates between a slower and faster pace— working at a high-intensity level for a designated amount of time, followed by a recovery period at a lower intensity. You can do HIIT with any aerobic activity—walking, running, biking, elliptical, swimming, rowing, etc.

The optimal ratio of high to low intensity is 1:3. For example, you work at your highest capacity of effort for 30 seconds, followed by a slower pace for 90 seconds. You could start out with a ten-minute workout made up of five intervals, alternating between running for 30 seconds and walking for 90 seconds.

Some additional tips:

- Warm up for at least three minutes.

- If you are just starting to exercise, start slow, with 15 seconds of high intensity and 45 seconds of low intensity, and just two or three sets of intervals. Work your way up one interval every two weeks, up to six to eight intervals. You can gradually increase the duration and intensity of your bursts.

- Don't overdo it. Keep interval training to 10- to 20-minute sessions and take a day off between HIIT training.

- Eat a healthy, balanced meal after exercise to rebuild and restore your body.

- Challenge your body by changing the types of exercise you do.

- Consult with your doctor before you start an exercise program, especially if you have any medical problems.

Strategies to Beat the Dreaded Plateau

A common complaint from those who are either trying to lose weight or become more fit is being stuck in a plateau. Below are some ways to get over the hump:

- Studies show intermittent fasting helps with both weight loss and longevity. One way to practice intermittent fasting is to significantly restrict calories (less than 500) for a period of 24 hours once per week. Fasting on workout days is not recommended. Another option is to fast for 12 hours between dinner and breakfast.

- Start with a five-minute aerobic warm-up, followed by a strength training routine, and ending your workout with HIIT. There is some evidence that this approach may promote fat loss.

- Exercise in the morning before breakfast. Studies show that twice as much fat is lost when exercise takes place in a fasting state.

- Be sure to have lots of water before your workout, and it's important to eat a balanced meal within 30 minutes after exercise. This should consist of high-quality protein, complex carbohydrates, and healthy fats.

- Consume a high-quality protein drink during exercise (20 grams whey protein, 3 ounces fresh-squeezed orange juice, and 1 tablespoon of raw honey) starting ten minutes into your workout.

Resistance Training—If You Don't Use It, You'll Lose It

"Resistance training" simply means working against resistance, which is very important to maintain your bone health and muscle strength. Many women avoid resistance training because they're afraid of "bulking up." However, if done correctly and in moderation, it won't make you overly muscular, but rather, will help you to be lean and toned. Simple resistance workouts use your body weight in exercises like squats, push-ups, pull-ups, and sit-ups.

Core Training

These exercises are designed to strengthen all the muscles around your trunk, including your abdominal muscles and the muscles of your back. Strengthening these muscles will not only help you look good, but it is very important for balance, as well as prevention of back pain. Pilates is a specific exercise routine that targets the muscles in your torso. You can also strengthen your core by exercising under conditions that require balance, like doing your exercises on an exercise ball.

The simplest core exercise is the "plank" hold, also called a "front hold," "hover," or "abdominal bridge." It calls for maintaining your body in a push-up position with the body's weight borne on the forearms, elbows, and toes for a period of time. Start with 15 seconds and work your way up to a minute or two.

Stretching

While this is one of the most neglected components of exercise, stretching is extremely important for overall wellness. Some of the many benefits of stretching include improved flexibility, circulation, and posture, as well as a decreased risk of muscle tension and soreness. As we age, we tend to lose flexibility, and stretching helps prevent the loss. Stretching should be done after warming up, or at the end of your workout program. Hold stretches for 15–60 seconds.

CHAPTER NINE

STEP SIX: HARNESS THE POWER OF SUNSHINE

Where there is sunshine, the doctor starves.

~ Flemish proverb

The numerous benefits of sunshine are well known, but the mechanism is not completely understood. Sunshine lowers blood pressure, alleviates depression, and improves skin conditions such as psoriasis. Daytime sun exposure also benefits your circadian rhythms by signaling your body that it is time to be awake.

It is not clear whether the benefits of sun exposure can all be attributed to the production of vitamin D, which the skin produces when exposed to it. However, the benefits of vitamin D are well studied and a deficiency is clearly a risk factor for many diseases.

News Flash: Vitamin D is not a Vitamin

An unfortunate misnomer, vitamin D is actually not a vitamin. It is a powerful hormone that your skin produces in response to sun exposure and affects over 2,000 genes and at least 36 organs of your body. With this widespread influence, it makes sense that vitamin D has a significant effect on your health. Vitamin D deficiency is associated with just about every chronic disease, most notably obesity, diabetes, hypertension, heart disease, cancer, osteoporosis, Alzheimer's disease, MS, migraines, asthma, and allergies.

While the primary source of vitamin D is the sun, you get a much smaller amount of vitamin D from the food you eat, primarily fatty fish and organ meats. Most people believe milk is a good source of this important hormone, but the D_2 form of the hormone artificially added to most milk is not the best form. As an example of how efficient your body is at synthesizing vitamin D, you make 10,000–20,000 IU of vitamin D after only 10–15 minutes of sunshine. An 8-ounce glass of milk only contains 100 IU, and multivitamins and calcium supplements contain only 400–1,000 IU.

Why Are We Deficient?

Fear of the sun, combined with our spending more time indoors in front of our electronics, has contributed to a widespread deficiency of this essential hormone. People are sun-phobic, either avoiding the sun or applying sunscreen prior to any exposure to prevent skin cancer. Sunscreen blocks vitamin D production. While sunburns and prolonged sun exposure can increase your risk for skin cancer, there is a certain type of skin cancer associated with vitamin D deficiency—basal cell carcinoma. Ironically, the sun can protect against this type of skin cancer.

Even those who spend time in the sun uncovered can be deficient because as we age, our skin is not as effective at converting sunshine into vitamin D. Although vitamin D deficiency is more common in northern regions of the world, it is still common in sunny areas. In my practice in St. Petersburg, Florida, approximately 70 percent of my patients have less than optimal levels of vitamin D.[148]

Benefits of Vitamin D

Unfortunately, a vitamin D blood level is usually not included as part of a routine physical. A thorough review of the research showing widespread benefits of vitamin D is beyond the scope of this book, but a 2015 article in a Harvard Public School of Health online publication provides a summary of recent research.[149] It summarizes vitamin D deficiency as a risk factor in heart attacks, heart failure, sudden cardiac death, stroke, many types of cancer, osteoporosis, autoimmune disease, depression, falls in the elderly, and infections, like the common cold and flu viruses. Isn't this enough evidence to screen everyone for vitamin D deficiency?

The media hasn't helped the case for vitamin D. In 2011, I received many calls from patients asking if they should stop their vitamin D supplements after there was an article in our local paper giving vitamin D a "thumbs down". The headline was deceiving because it only reported on a panel review by the Institute of Medicine to update the recommended daily allowance (RDA) for vitamin D.[150] The committee increased the RDA to 600 IU for children and adults and 800 IU for those over the age of 71, but concluded that further research is necessary before recommending a higher RDA for everyone. They did not comment on blood levels of vitamin D or treating a deficiency, stating that such a deficiency was not widespread and that most people get enough from sunshine and food.

A second article, again giving a "thumbs down" to vitamin D, was based on another panel recommendation from the US Preventive Task Force.[151] They said that women shouldn't take vitamin D to prevent fractures because vitamin D at the typical doses in calcium supplements (400 IU) doesn't prevent fractures.[152] These panel recommendations do not, in any way, address the problem of vitamin D deficiency. By presenting information in a sensationalized way in order to create interesting headlines, the media contributes to the confusion.

It should have been the actual studies that got the "thumbs down" for poor design, rather than vitamin D taking the hit. A summary of the evidence from 12 fracture trials that included more than 40,000 people found that a moderate dosage of vitamin D (about 800 IU per day) reduced hip and non-spine fractures by 20 percent, while lower intake (400 IU or less) failed to offer any benefit.[153] Vitamin D also reduces the risk of falls by 20 percent in the elderly, but only if taken in higher doses (700 to 1,000 IU).[154]

Studies have shown a decrease in prevalence of some cancers, diabetes, multiple sclerosis, and fractures when vitamin D blood levels are in the range of 40-60 ng/mL.[155, 156,157,158,159] Further well-designed research studies are being conducted to determine the optimal blood levels of vitamin D, as well as the impact of correcting vitamin D deficiency on disease.

The form of vitamin D supplement taken is also important. Vitamin D_3 shows superiority, being more effective at raising blood levels and also better converted to the active form in the body than vitamin D_2. The D_3 form also lasts longer in the body and has a longer shelf life.[160, 161, 162, 163, 164] The form prescribed by doctors is often inferior D_2.

Vitamin D Facts & Tips

- To get optimal levels of sun exposure, you should spend 10–15 minutes per day outside, preferably at peak hours, before applying sunscreen.

- If you take a supplement, make sure it is in the form of vitamin D_3 (cholecalciferol), not vitamin D_2 (ergocalciferol).

- You can have your level checked with an inexpensive blood test. The preferred vitamin D test is the 25-OH vitamin D blood test.

- Do not take high doses (more than 2,000 IU daily) unless you are having levels monitored. Vitamin D can increase to toxic levels with prolonged high-dose supplementation.

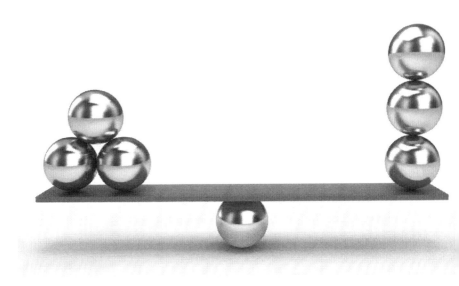

CHAPTER TEN

STEP SEVEN: ACHIEVE HORMONE BALANCE

Most of us are living life completely out of balance. But so many symptoms we come to accept as "normal" are just signs of imbalance—and the type of imbalance that affects almost everyone in our society is hormonal imbalance.

~ Mark Hyman, MD

Road Map to Health: 7 Steps to Alter Your Destination

A "Symphony of Hormones"

Hormone balance and dysfunction are concepts people have a hard time grasping because the endocrine system is very complex. Hormones are the chemicals that allow different parts of your body to communicate with each other. If any of these hormones are unbalanced, it can have far-reaching effects on the body. It's like a symphony, with each hormone being a different instrument. When one instrument is out of tune, the song just doesn't sound right. And similarly, when one hormone is out of balance, the whole body just doesn't function right.

Conventional medicine often approaches hormone balance from the wrong direction, treating the problem at the end of a cascade of events, rather than at the beginning. This "downstream" method of treating problems, rather than looking "upstream" at what caused the dysfunction in the first place, does not honor the body as a whole system.

A Functional Medicine approach takes into consideration the complex interplay of the endocrine system in health and disease. It's important to approach hormonal imbalance in a specific way, addressing the root cause of the dysfunction.

The first step is to look at the health of the gut, the center of the body's universe, so to speak (see Chapter 3). An unhealthy gut can lead to widespread hormone imbalance. The next focus should be on adrenal function, which has the widest effect on the rest of the system. Thyroid and reproductive hormones should be addressed last because they often come back into balance with correction of the gut and/or adrenals.

Hormones 101

A basic understanding of the endocrine system is important in order to understand the repercussions of imbalance. The hormone-producing organs that make up our endocrine system include parts of our brain (hypothalamus, pituitary, and pineal glands), thyroid and parathyroid glands, adrenal glands, thymus, pancreas, and reproductive organs (ovaries in women and testes in men). Cholesterol is the building block for all our adrenal and reproductive hormones and they are closely intertwined. Adrenal hormones also have significant effects on thyroid and pancreatic hormones.

The Center of the Endocrine System—Adrenal Glands

The adrenals are at the center of the symphony, producing the hormone DHEA, which is the precursor of both our cortisol and reproductive hormones. The adrenals drive the production of cortisol, the primary stress hormone that produces the fight-or-flight response discussed in the last chapter. When your body is constantly in a fight-or-flight mode, you need to produce more cortisol, at the expense of your reproductive hormones (see Figure 1). This is probably the reason why stress can cause menstrual periods to stop in young women. In addition, a study from the Boston University analyzed the cases of 600 women between the ages of 36 and 45 and found that women under chronic stress are 80 percent more likely to experience early menopause.[165] In my practice, I have also observed a connection between stress and the severity of menopausal symptoms.

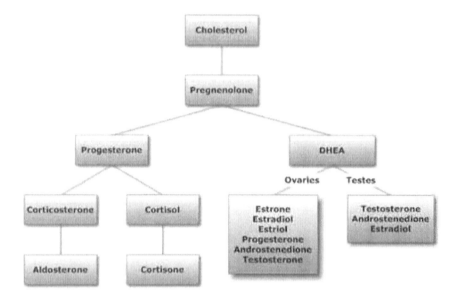

Figure 1[166]

The Sugar Manager—Pancreas

Although the pancreas is not an organ that most people are familiar with, the primary hormone of the pancreas is at the root of the serious epidemic of diabetes and obesity. The pancreas releases insulin in response to surges in blood sugar levels. When we eat a lot of carbohydrates in the form of sugar and starches, especially those quickly absorbed carbohydrates in highly processed foods, our pancreas responds by releasing insulin in order to let this sugar into the cells. A common misconception is that diabetes is only associated with candy and other sweets. There are many non-sweet foods that are just as bad, if not worse, for your blood sugar—bread, pasta, crackers, and chips, to name a few.

When insulin levels are always high, our cells need more and more insulin to have the same effect. This is called "insulin resistance" and is a risk factor for future diabetes. When cells become resistant to insulin, a

high level of insulin is required to keep your blood sugar in a
ely normal range. At this stage, your doctor may tell you that your
d sugar level is normal, but unknown to you, the high insulin level is
eaking havoc all over your body, promoting inflammation and plaque
buildup in the arteries.[167] It also promotes storage of visceral fat ("belly
fat") and weight gain. This is why the types of foods we eat, rather than
just the calories, affect whether or not we will become fat. Insulin
resistance needs to be detected before the blood sugar is elevated. A
fasting blood insulin level is the best way to determine insulin
resistance.

Conventional medicine waits until there is a "disease" to take action.
Have you ever been told your blood sugar was "a little high,"
"borderline," or that you have "pre-diabetes?" What does this mean,
and what do you need to do about it? Pre-diabetes means that your
blood sugar is above normal, but not high enough to meet the cut-off
for diabetes. At this stage, your doctor will probably give you a vague
recommendation to "exercise, eat right, and lose weight," but reassure
you that you don't have diabetes. Doctors often pay little attention until
you actually do have diabetes, and then will prescribe medication to
lower your blood sugar.

The sad part is that the easiest time to reverse this process is at the first
sign of insulin resistance—before blood sugar is elevated. The damage
from high insulin levels starts years—probably even decades—earlier,
before your blood sugar is even in the pre-diabetic range. Diabetes
causes blindness, kidney failure, nerve damage, heart attacks, stroke,
and increases risk for depression, cancer, and dementia. Below are the
values I use in my practice.

Level	Fasting Insulin	Fasting Blood Sugar
Optimal	<6	<87
Suboptimal	6–10	88–99
Pre-diabetes	>10	100–125
Diabetes	Variable	>126

The bottom line is that the choices you make each day determine the development of insulin resistance and, ultimately, diabetes—the choice to eat processed food, avoid exercise, stay up late, and/or ignore chronic stress. The only treatment that addresses the root cause of the problem is a change in lifestyle, especially what you choose to eat every day.

The Body's Thermostat—Thyroid

Acting like your body's automatic thermostat, the thyroid adjusts your metabolism based on ambient conditions and is very sensitive to the balance of the entire system. For example, when you're ill, your body needs to slow metabolism so it can use its energy to recover. Thyroid dysfunction is often over-treated with medication; I see patients who were started on thyroid medication after one single blood test came back slightly out of range. One of the thyroid hormones, TSH, can sometimes be out of range, especially during illness, and then is normal when rechecked.

Many factors can lead to a sluggish thyroid, including chronic stress or nutritional deficiencies. A number of nutrients are needed by the

/roid to produce thyroid hormone, including iodine, selenium, and B ,tamins. Another factor that can cause thyroid dysfunction includes chemicals in food, specifically the endocrine-disrupting chemicals (EDCs) discussed in previous chapters. Food sensitivities, especially gluten, are associated with autoimmune thyroid disease. Simply putting somebody on a thyroid medication is often not the best solution. The focus should be on addressing the underlying problem to see if the thyroid corrects itself.

Thyroid dysfunction can also be underdiagnosed in two ways: First, doctors most often just check a TSH level, which doesn't give a complete picture of thyroid function. TSH is the hormone produced by the pituitary gland in the brain that tells the thyroid gland to produce free T_4. Relying on TSH alone can miss thyroid dysfunction. Free T_4 is converted to free T_3, the active thyroid hormone. It is very important to check both thyroid hormones, free T_3 and free T_4, as some people have inadequate conversion of free T_4 to free T_3.

Comprehensive blood testing to evaluate the thyroid includes thyroid antibodies (to detect autoimmune thyroid disease), TSH, free T_4, free T_3, and reverse T_3. It is especially important to check reverse T_3 because it is like the "brake" for the thyroid, blocking the active thyroid hormone, free T_3, in order to slow down the thyroid's activity. When elevated, reverse T_3 can cause a hypothyroid state, even in the presence of normal levels of thyroid hormones.

Second, the normal reference range for thyroid labs is much too wide, missing a diagnosis in many patients. Having the same reference range for everyone is like saying we all should wear the same size shoe. It is important to consider patients' symptoms as well as the results of the appropriate testing.

Fertility & Sex—Testes & Ovaries

The reproductive hormones progesterone, estrogen, and testosterone are produced by the adrenal gland, testes, and ovaries. All of these hormones are produced in both men and women, albeit in different amounts. Imbalance of the reproductive hormones is affected by all of the factors I have described in this book, including poor diet, lack of exercise, stress, lack of sleep, and exposure to EDCs.

Some of the EDCs mentioned in Chapter 5 imitate estrogen in the body and are called "xeno-estrogens," which means "foreign estrogen." Exposure to these chemicals increases overall estrogen activity in the body, referred to as "estrogen dominance." Exposure to xeno-estrogens happens every day, with some of the more common sources being plastics, air fresheners, household cleaners, non-organic dairy and meats, pesticides, sunscreens, skin care products, and dry cleaning chemicals.

This is particularly important to note by people who have a history or family history of diseases linked to estrogen excess—in women, uterine fibroids (benign growths in the uterus), breast cysts, breast cancer, migraines, and endometriosis. Estrogen dominance in men is linked to infertility, erectile dysfunction, prostate enlargement, and prostate cancer. If you have any history or family history of these problems, it is very important to reduce your exposure to these chemicals. Even more concerning, the problem of xeno-estrogens is a journey into the unknown for our children and their future health.

Other Important "Players"

Other organs of the body produce hormones as well. When exposed to adequate sunlight, the skin produces vitamin D. Remember that vitamin D is not a vitamin, but a powerful hormone affecting every part of your body. Cells in the gut also produce several hormones that affect appetite, digestion, and movement of food through the gastrointestinal tract. The kidneys produce hormones that produce red blood cells, help convert vitamin D to its active form, and regulate blood pressure. The heart even produces its own hormones to help control blood pressure. Furthermore, the balance or imbalance of these hormones has an intricate interplay with each other.

Hormone Replacement Therapy

As men and women age, many suffer from symptoms caused by decreasing levels of reproductive hormones. As mentioned earlier, poor diet and inflammation, stress, exposure to chemicals, and lack of exercise and sleep all contribute to hormone imbalance in men and women. Changes in lifestyle should be the primary focus of restoring the balance of reproductive hormones.

Some patients have symptoms despite changes in lifestyle and may benefit from supplementing with hormones, a treatment referred to as Hormone Replacement Therapy (HRT). Most people are familiar with the common menopausal symptoms of mood swings, hot flashes, and night sweats. But women and men can also suffer from difficulty concentrating, decreased libido and sexual dysfunction, poor sleep, depression and irritability, weight gain, and loss of muscle and bone strength. Correcting hormone levels with hormone replacement can improve these symptoms and quality of life as we age.

Bioidentical versus Synthetic

The idea of replacing deficient hormones in women suffering from menopausal symptoms is not a new idea. Records dating back to the 11th century report that Chinese physicians used dried crystalized urine from younger women to help aging women with the symptoms associated with menopause.

A lot of confusion about synthetic versus bioidentical hormones exists. Bioidentical simply means the hormone is identical to the hormones produced in the human body. Bioidentical hormones used today are derived from soybeans and wild yams, which contain a compound with the same basic chemical structure as human hormones. It still needs to be converted to estradiol, progesterone, or testosterone in a laboratory. These compounds are natural in the sense that they are derived from plants and are identical to your own body's hormones.

Hormones that are not bioidentical affect the same receptors, but they are not identical to what your body produces. The most well-known non-bioidentical hormone is Premarin, which is made from the urine of pregnant horses. This estrogen-like drug is not identical to human estrogen (more on Premarin in a minute).

"Big Pharma" versus "Little Pharma"

Bioidentical hormones are used by both pharmaceutical companies and compounding pharmacies to make bioidentical hormone preparations. The difference is that pharmaceutical companies, with the goal of making mass-produced drugs that generate big profits, create patented delivery systems for both synthetic and bioidentical hormones.

Despite what many people think, bioidentical hormones are available at retail pharmacies. The most commonly used bioidentical estrogen, estradiol, is available at various dose levels in pill, patch, cream, and gel forms. Progesterone is also available at retail pharmacies in oral form as generic progesterone and the brand version, Prometrium.

Compounding pharmacies are independent pharmacies that "compound" or formulate medications for individual patients. They use the same bioidentical hormones to make individualized formulas for each patient based on the doctor's prescribed dosage. So another difference between retail and compounding pharmacies is that retail pharmacies have a limited number of dosing options as opposed to compounding pharmacies, whose dosing options are limitless.

Compounding pharmacies have attracted a lot of criticism from the conventional medicine community. Although the individual medications used by compounding pharmacies are approved for use in the US, the formulations are not FDA approved. The regulation of compounding pharmacies falls to each individual state. There is concern that without central FDA regulation, there are inadequate checks and balances of the quality of compounded medications.

In October 2012, a meningitis outbreak resulted in 64 deaths from a contaminated, injectable medication made by a single compounding pharmacy located in Massachusetts.[168] Individual states came under enormous pressure to regulate compounding pharmacies after this tragic outbreak. Regulation efforts by the federal government led to passage of the Drug Quality and Security Act in 2013, which encourages compounding pharmacies to register with the FDA. If a compounding pharmacy registers with the FDA, hospitals and other health-care providers will be able to buy their products.

The compounding pharmacy industry has also made efforts at self-regulation. Those that have attained accreditation by the Pharmacy Compounding Accreditation Board (PCAB) must comply with inspections and strict quality requirements.

History of HRT in Women

In the 1950s, the pharmaceutical industry saw an opportunity to create patented synthetic hormones since patented drugs can generate huge profits. They started advertising, to women and physicians, a new treatment for the aging female. Through a well-strategized marketing campaign, they created the disease of menopause and the treatments, their estrogen-like drug, Premarin, and Provera, a synthetic progesterone-like hormone not identical to human progesterone. The combination of the two drugs, Prempro, became the bestselling drug in the US. In 2001, it generated a record-breaking profit of $2 billion for the drug company Wyeth.

In 2002, the Women's Health Initiative study was published. This large analysis, following 160,000 women over eight years, indicated that the risks of taking oral Prempro outweighed the benefits received. Although the drug reduced bone fractures and colon cancer, there were other, more significant consequences, including blood clots, breast cancer, heart attacks, and strokes.[169] Panicked doctors immediately began taking patients off Premarin and Prempro. Predictably, these women started to feel horrible after the sudden discontinuation. Their physicians told them there were no alternatives and instead prescribed antidepressants or birth control pills—with poor results and unpleasant side effects.

Since that time, conventional medicine has ignored the effectiveness of bioidentical hormone therapy (BHRT) as an option. Hundreds of studies in the US and Europe over the past 25 years have demonstrated that bioidentical hormones, estradiol and progesterone, are equally or more effective than hormones that are not bioidentical—and also safer.[170, 171] Yet, mainstream medicine, strongly influenced by the pharmaceutical industry, refuses to take these studies seriously. Furthermore, due to the drug companies' strong influence on medical education, most doctors are not educated about bioidentical hormones or the way in which different hormone molecules work.

While Europeans have used bioidentical hormones for quite some time, the FDA had been slow to approve them until 1998, when a few

Stacey J. Robinson, MD

pharmaceutical companies obtained FDA approval for an array of bioidentical estrogen preparations (estradiol) and one progesterone preparation. The pharmaceutical companies still generate huge profits by patenting the delivery method, creating different types of patches and gels.

Despite the lack of acceptance of individualized BHRT in conventional medicine, women have discovered—on their own—the convenience and flexibility of compounding pharmacies that are able to create individually prepared bioidentical hormones in a variety of forms (oral capsules, creams, gels, oils, and sublingual tablets in the exact dosage the doctor prescribes.

HRT in Men

Testosterone replacement in men isn't quite as complex, since all the available testosterone preparations are bioidentical. The only difference is the delivery method, which can be in the form of topical creams and gels, troches, injections, and implantable pellets (more on this below).

Concerns have been raised about the possible risks of prostate cancer and heart attacks in men treated with testosterone. The possible link between testosterone replacement and heart attacks was contradicted by larger, better designed studies which demonstrated that correcting low testosterone actually improves many cardiac risk markers, including cholesterol, blood sugar, blood pressure, and inflammation.[172]

Furthermore, a 2015 Mayo Clinic report summarized all the research to date on testosterone replacement and heart attack risk and declared there is no increased risk of heart attack with testosterone replacement. Instead, it appears to be protective.[173] Similarly, a review of all the literature on prostate cancer and testosterone therapy has not shown any increased risk.[174, 175]

When we talk about risks, it is important to note we are talking about correcting testosterone levels in men who have low levels, but there is some controversy about the definition of "low" testosterone. I think everyone would agree that a level below 300 ng/dL is low. In my opinion, levels between 300–550 ng/dL are relatively low, and levels between 550–900 ng/dL would be considered normal to optimal. It is important to take into consideration the age of the patient, since testosterone levels do decline with age, as well as whether or not the patient has symptoms consistent with low testosterone such as decreased libido, fatigue, difficulty concentrating, poor sleep, depressed mood, and loss of muscle strength. The level at which a man will have symptoms will vary from person to person, so once again, it shouldn't be a "one size fits all" treatment.

When prescribing testosterone replacement, it is very important to check estrogen levels. Testosterone is converted to estrogen in the body, and this conversion varies from person to person. If estradiol levels are too high, it may result in more estrogen-linked disease, as discussed earlier. If the levels are high, a medication to block the conversion (aromatase inhibitor) should also be prescribed.

Delivery Methods

As mentioned, BHRT can be delivered by many different routes. The difference between the various delivery methods is their very different availability patterns.

Troches are the quickest to act (within hours) and shorter acting, so they require twice-daily dosing. Creams have a slower onset and last a little longer, usually requiring daily dosing. Injections of testosterone are of slower onset and longer duration, so injections are needed every one to three weeks.

Pellets, which are inserted under the skin by a health-care practitioner, are the only form of delivery that mirrors how ovaries and testicles produce hormone levels in steady, around-the-clock low dosages. Pellets last, on average, three months for women and six months for men. Made by compounding pharmacies, dosages are more precise than other methods and are determined individually by your blood hormone levels as well as other factors.

I have prescribed all forms of BHRT to patients for many years. My preferred delivery method for safety and convenience is either topical applications or pellets. The downside of topical hormones is that they are more difficult to get steady, adequate levels. My experience is that patients don't see as much symptomatic improvement.

With pellets, it is much easier to achieve adequate levels and patients report much more symptom improvement in sexual function, sleep, energy, mood, exercise ability, and increase in muscle and loss of fat. The downsides to pellets are temporary soreness or itching at the insertion site in some patients, and about a 10 percent chance that one or more pellets will come out from the site (extrusion), which can be a nuisance. Also, pellets can't easily be removed, so in the rare case that the patient has a side effect, they have to wait a few months until the pellets dissolve for the side effect to go away.

Mary's Story

After menopause, many women suffer from atrophic vaginitis, a thinning of the vaginal lining that causes dryness and, in some cases, very painful intercourse. When I first met Mary, this problem was first on her list of concerns because it was having a significant effect on her relationship with her husband. She had been through menopause about ten years prior and had suffered from vaginal dryness and painful intercourse ever since. She tried many different topical hormone preparations, but none offered any improvement.

Upon further discussion, she also complained of low libido, fatigue, depressed mood, and poor sleep. Both her estrogen and testosterone blood levels were very low. Interestingly, although she had severe atrophic vaginitis, she did not complain of the typical hot flashes that most women experience with low estrogen levels.

She decided to try pellet therapy with estrogen and testosterone. Within a few months, she reported more energy, better mood, and her long-departed libido had finally returned. After years of restless sleep, she was also "sleeping like a baby." Most importantly, the vaginal pain was almost completely resolved and she was able to enjoy sex with her husband again. This demonstrates how a simple treatment can have profound effects on a person's quality of life.

PART III—PUTTING IT ALL TOGETHER

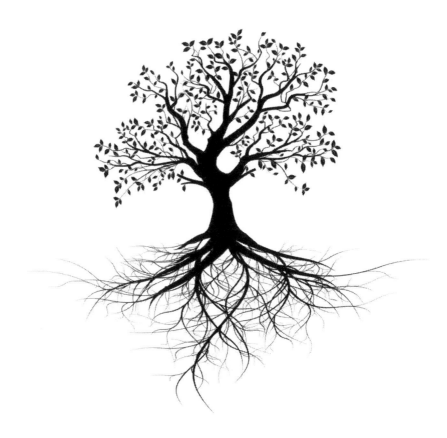

CHAPTER ELEVEN

CHOOSING HEALTH OVER DISEASE

Motivation is what gets you started. Habit is what keeps you going.

~ Jim Ryun, Olympic Medalist

The decision to become healthier is a choice. Are you happy with the status quo? Often we know we want to change and we know what we have to do. We just can't get motivated to take action.

The one pill I wish Big Pharma would formulate is a motivation pill. The word "motivation" is derived from the verb "motivate," which means "to move." It is the fire within us that determines whether we will take action, and it can sometimes be elusive. The first step is to sit down and contemplate the factors involved in your decision to act or not to act.

What factors play into your decision to take action? Most influential is our "why"—the internal beliefs that shape our choices. Do you believe that food, movement, and rest/relaxation determine your long-term health? What impact would better health have on your life?

Make a list of all the reasons you should make these changes. Then, for each reason, ask yourself why you want the change. And keep asking yourself why until you get as deep as possible.

Once you determine your "why" and you believe, deep in your heart, that a change is going to affect you in a positive way, then you need to ask yourself, "What is holding me back?" These are the reasons or obstacles that keep you from making a change. Then I would challenge you to do the following:

1) Ask yourself if your excuse is true and valid. You really don't have time to exercise? You can't take 15 minutes out of your 24-hour day? That leaves you 23 hours and 45 minutes to do everything else. "I don't have time" is probably the most common excuse I hear, and it is probably the weakest excuse. We all make time for what is important.

2) If your excuse is true, view it as a problem that needs a solution. If you find exercise boring, ask yourself if there is any activity that inv moving your body that you enjoy. Exercise doesn't have to mear to the gym and running on a treadmill or working out on weight machines. You can garden or take a dance class, join a sports team, explore local walking trails, or help your busy friends walk their dogs.

I have discovered over the years that the more I learn, the more I want to move toward living a healthier lifestyle. There are so many people around you who can help you to learn. Explore restaurants and markets in your area that provide healthy food. Read blogs and books and watch movies about living healthier. You will find that gradually, you will gain a deep desire to change. But keep in mind that change doesn't happen overnight.

Check out the Resources at the end of this book. Choose one book to read or movie to watch next. My goal in writing this book is to fuel your beliefs about the powerful impact nutrition, movement, and rest/relaxation can have on your health. I also want to reduce your obstacles by showing you that it is not as complicated as you think. Healthy living is actually quite simple once you have the information and tools to make healthy choices.

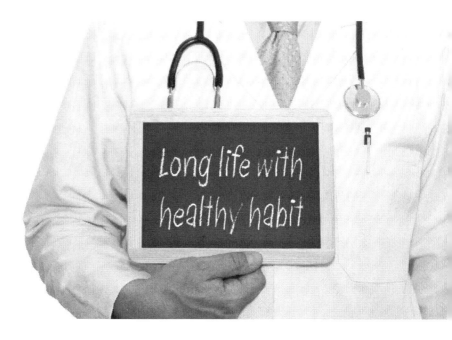

CHAPTER TWELVE

HOW TO CREATE HABITS THAT STICK

We are what we repeatedly do. Excellence, then, is not an act, but a habit.

~ Aristotle

In order to alter your daily behaviors, it's important to first understand your habits. According to Merriam Webster, a "habit" is something that a person does, often in a regular and repeated way. It is also something that can be hard to give up. Wouldn't you like to come to the point where exercise, eating healthy, and spending time relaxing are activities that would be hard for you NOT to do? The answer, of course, is likely to be a resounding "YES!" I think we all want to have easy, healthy habits that we want to do each day.

All habits have a three-step pattern proven by researchers in the world of behavior psychology. First there is a reminder or cue, then a routine (the habit itself), and third, a consequence. If the consequence is positive, you will want to repeat the routine.

The following are some steps from James Clear, author of *Transform Your Habits that* you can use to transform the routine described in the next chapter into a habit.

1) Set a reminder. Pick something you do, or something that happens to you, each day without fail and use it as a reminder for your new behavior. For example, if having coffee or tea is part of your morning routine, then practice your meditation or controlled breathing right after you have a cup of coffee or tea. Reminders are critical because it takes a minimum of two months for behaviors to become habits.

2) Be sure to choose a habit that is easy to start, and start small. It's all about small steps that eventually create big change. If you don't exercise at all, then start by taking a ten-minute walk. Don't start by going to the gym for a 90-minute workout.

3) Reward yourself. Many healthy habits have inherent rewards. When you exercise, you usually feel better and have more energy. You may lose weight, which is rewarding in itself. But if the behavior doesn't have positive effect immediately, be sure to give yourself a reward, even if it is just telling yourself, "Great job exercising today!" Or you can anticipate a bigger reward, such as buying yourself a new outfit after you have exercised every day for a week.

Road Map to Health: 7 Steps to Alter Your Destination

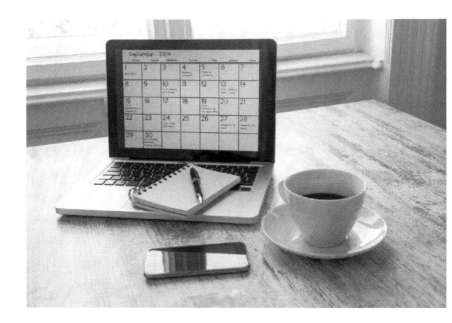

CHAPTER THIRTEEN

THESE SIMPLE DAILY HABITS WILL TRANSFORM

YOUR HEALTH

The best time to plant a tree was 20 years ago. The next best time is now.

~ Chinese Proverb

What's stopping you from making changes today? It's all about the small lifestyle choices you make every single day that move you in a certain trajectory toward your future health. Your genes are not always your destiny. Your daily choices change the way your genes are expressed.

Remember, conventional medicine waits until disease happens and then throws meds at it, calling that "doctoring." Only that isn't doctoring—not the right kind, anyway. You can doctor yourself and achieve better results with the following routine.

Eight Elements that Must be Part of Your Daily Routine

1) Breathe. Start and end your day with controlled breathing, yoga, or meditation. If you don't yet meditate or practice yoga, simply start with five minutes of the 4-7-8 controlled breath exercise (see Chapter 6). Also, do the 4-7-8 exercise anytime you feel anxiety or muscle tension from stressors. Once you master controlled breathing, consider joining a yoga class or taking a meditation course.

2) Hydrate. Drink a glass of water as soon as you wake up. Your body is 60 percent water and water helps to cleanse and filter the toxins out of your system. Drink water throughout the day and eliminate unhealthy beverages like sodas and sweetened or artificially sweetened drinks. Add the juice of ½ a lemon to your water, giving you a good boost of vitamin C.

3) Move. If you don't currently exercise, start simply walking ten minutes each morning, and then add some HIIT intervals. Move more throughout the day by taking the stairs and parking at the farthest spaces in the lot. If you already exercise, make sure you are practicing all components—cardio with intervals, resistance training, core strengthening, and stretching. Consider working with a personal trainer for motivation and guidance on how to change your workout to challenge your body.

4) Get sunshine. Expose yourself to the sun for at least ten minutes per day. Take your daily walk outside in the sunshine, or take a 15-minute break from work and go outside for fresh air and sunshine. Get your vitamin D level checked and take a supplement if needed.

5) Be positive. Strive to have a positive attitude every day. Make a gratitude list and refer to it daily. Forgive your enemies for your own benefit. Let go of the circumstances and people that you can't control. Find your passion and connect with others who share it. Surround yourself with positive people who lift you up.

6) Relax. Take at least 15 minutes each day for an activity such as listening to relaxing music, meditating, controlled breathing, yoga, Tai Chi, laughing, or praying. These endeavors will decrease the impact of stress, which promotes aging and disease.

7) Fuel your body. You are what you eat, so make it count! Take control of what you put in your body by preparing your food or eating at restaurants that offer clean, whole foods. Read Chapter 5 again and remember that food is the most powerful medicine. Pick one of the eight steps outlined and start today. End each day with a plan for what you will eat the following day. Assemble some Overnight Oats and Salad in a Jar (see Chapter 14) for your breakfast and lunch the next day. Pack healthy snacks to have with you so you aren't tempted to raid the vending machine at work.

8) Sleep. Get seven to eight hours of sleep per night. Go through the sleep checklist to ensure you are helping your body get the time it needs for rest and repair to slow the aging process. Go to bed earlier—it really is "beauty rest."

So whether you're healthy, have symptoms of imbalance, or have already been diagnosed with a chronic disease, the daily routine listed above can help move you toward better health. It addresses stress, a sedentary lifestyle, and poor diet—our biggest enemies, killing us slowly by accelerating disease and aging.

The body's natural healing mechanism is so much more powerful than any medication I could ever prescribe. It is such a complex system we will never be able to fully understand it. But while the body is complex, the way it should be cared for is quite simple.

The bottom line is that our body often has the power to rebalance and heal itself—if you provide what it needs: eat real, clean food; move every day; rest and relax; and be positive.

I would like to join you on your journey to optimal health. For continued motivation, go to my website, RobinsonMed.com, and sign up for my health tips. Also be sure to connect with me on my RobinsonMed Facebook page and follow me on Twitter @StaceyRMD.

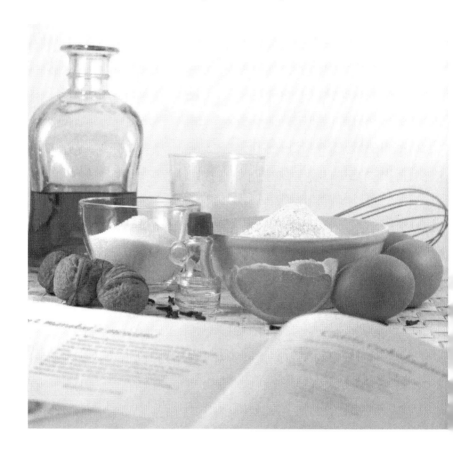

CHAPTER FOURTEEN

RECIPES: YOUR PRESCRIPTION FOR HEALTH

The fork is your most powerful tool to change your health.

~ Mark Hyman, MD

This chapter provides a few simple, easy-to-prepare recipes that can be the mainstay of your routine. One of the most difficult obstacles I have found in my practice is helping people who aren't confident with or accustomed to cooking and preparing meals.

Preparing food is not difficult, but is one of the most important tools you can have in eating a clean diet. Once you learn some basic skills, I encourage you to find recipes online, or in cookbooks, and experiment.

Breakfast Smoothie

Ingredients

- 1 cup mixed frozen berries
- ½ banana
- 1 cup almond or coconut milk
- ½ cup orange juice
- 2 cups kale or other greens
- 2 tbsp ground chia or flax
- 1–2 scoops high-quality rice/pea protein

Directions

Combine all ingredients in a blender or food processor. Add water and ice to desired consistency. Refrigerate leftovers.

Weekday Vegetable Soup

Ingredients

- 1 yellow onion, chopped

- 2 celery stalks, diced
- 3 carrots, thinly sliced
- 1 garlic clove, minced
- 1 tsp paprika
- ⅛ tsp turmeric
- ½ tsp pepper
- 1 tsp salt (or to taste)
- 2–3 fresh tomatoes, chopped
- 4 cups organic vegetable broth
- 2 cans white, kidney, black, garbanzo, or other beans, drained and rinsed (make sure cans are BPA free)
- ½ cup quinoa or diced sweet potatoes (optional)
- 2–4 cups kale, spinach, collard, or other greens

Directions

Sauté first four ingredients in 1 tbsp of olive or coconut oil.

Add spices, vegetable broth, tomatoes, beans, and quinoa or sweet potatoes. Simmer for 20–30 minutes or until veggies/quinoa are tender.

You can blend one can beans in blender or food processor and add to the soup for a thicker consistency.

Five minutes before serving, add greens.

You can add more broth and/or water for desired consistency. Experiment with other veggies, herbs, and spices.

Salad in a Jar

Salad in a Jar is one of my favorite lunches. I assemble it after dinner from my leftovers and other ingredients in my fridge. It takes very little time and I have lunch ready to go in the morning. If you prepare before cleaning up from dinner, there is no separate cleanup required.

Assembling it in the correct order is important so the lettuce or other greens don't get soggy. Take it to work and simply shake it up and put it on a plate for a healthy lunch with lots of veggies, protein, and healthy fat. Be creative, with a variety of ingredients, so you don't get bored. Below is the basic recipe and some examples of how to mix things up.

Ingredients & Directions

In a large mason jar, assemble the following in the order shown:

Layer 1—Dressing—whisk together oil, vinegar, herbs, and spices

Layer 2—Hearty vegetables (chopped or sliced)

Layer 3—Beans and less hearty vegetables (chopped or sliced)

Layer 4—Protein (grilled, baked, or broiled)

Layer 5—Lettuce and/or greens (use any variety)

Layer 6—Cheese (optional)

Layer 7—Toasted nuts/seeds (toast in pan or broiler until golden)

See Variations on Next Page

	Wedge	Asian	Greek	Brussels Slaw
Healthy oil, 1 tsp	Olive oil	Sesame oil	Olive oil	Avocado oil
Vinegar or acid, 1 tbsp	Balsamic	Rice vinegar	Lemon juice	Cider vinegar
Other			Oregano, ½ tsp	Dijon mustard, 1 tsp
Veggie (layer 2)	Cucumbers Red or yellow bell peppers Red onion	Cucumbers Broccoli	Cucumbers Green bell pepper Red onion	Shallot
Veggie (layer 3)	Cherry tomatoes	Green onion	Roma tomatoes	
Protein	Chicken or steak	Chicken, shrimp, tofu, or edamame	Chick peas	Grated or chopped hard-boiled egg
Cheese	Blue Cheese		Feta	Parmesan
Lettuce	Iceberg/ Romaine	Butter lettuce	Romaine and spinach	Thinly sliced raw Brussels sprouts
Nuts or Seeds	Pumpkin seeds	Cashews and sesame seeds	Pine nuts	Almonds

Overnight Oats

There are several advantages of having Overnight Oats for breakfast—no cooking required, preparation occurs the night before, and they are healthy and delicious. A vast number of recipe combinations allow you to be creative.

Ingredients

- ½ cup rolled oats* (you can use steel cut oats, but they will be chewier)
- 2 tbsp ground chia or flax seed—this gives you a boost of healthy omega-3 fats
- 1 cup liquid—I prefer non-dairy milk, either coconut, almond, or cashew milk. You can use soy milk, but make sure it is organic/non-GMO (most soy in the US is GMO). You can also use 50:50 combinations of unsweetened yogurt and milk.
- Sweetener—honey, pure maple syrup, coconut sugar, brown sugar, raw cane sugar, or organic applesauce
- Spices—½–1 tsp
- Fruit—¼ cup
- Nuts—toasted and chopped or slivered are best. Toasted coconut is also delicious as a topping.

*If you have gluten sensitivity or want to be gluten free, make sure to buy gluten free oats. Oats do not contain gluten but are often contaminated in processing.

Directions

Mix the oats, chia or flax, milk, sweetener, and spices in a mason jar.

Place fruit and nuts on top. Seal and refrigerate overnight.

Variations

	Apple Pie	PB&J	Peaches & Cream
Spices/flavors	½ tsp cinnamon ¼ tsp vanilla ¼ tsp nutmeg	2 tbsp natural peanut or almond butter	½ tsp cinnamon
Liquid	coconut milk	almond milk	cashew milk
Fruit	½ apple—diced	raspberries or strawberries	peaches
Nuts	1 tbsp walnuts	none	pecans
Sweetener	2 tbsp applesauce	1 tbsp maple syrup	2 tbsp honey

Basic Vinaigrette

One of the most common sources of hidden sugars, GMO oils, and other additives/preservatives is bottled salad dressings. It is much healthier, not to mention less costly, to make your own.

Ingredients

- Oil—cold pressed, extra virgin olive, walnut, avocado, or sesame oil
- Vinegar—balsamic, red wine, or rice vinegar (lemon juice can also be used)
- Flavors—Dijon mustard, chopped anchovies, chopped tomatoes
- Herbs—chopped, fresh herbs are best, but you can also use dried herbs. The conversion of fresh to dry is 1 tbsp fresh equals 1 tsp dried.

Directions

Using a ratio of 2:1 oil to vinegar makes it easy to increase or decrease the amount you want to make. It is important to add a little sea salt to bring out the flavors.

If you like your salad dressing sweet, you can add a little honey to taste.

Oven Roasted Veggies

These will make a convert out of anyone who doesn't like vegetables. The flavors that come out with roasting are amazing, and you can roast just about any vegetable.

Ingredients & Directions

Place chopped veggies in a roasting pan. You can use any veggies, but my favorites are broccoli, cauliflower, green beans, zucchini/summer squash, mushrooms, and Brussels sprouts.

Add a handful of sliced raw garlic cloves.

Toss with 1 tbsp olive oil.

Sprinkle with freshly ground sea salt to taste.

Roast at 400° for 15–30 minutes or until tender and golden brown.

Healthy Snack Ideas

- Fresh fruit, such as berries, with plain yogurt and drizzle of honey
- A handful of nuts (best if raw and organic)
- Handful of trail mix with nuts, seeds, and dried fruit
- Slice of Swiss cheese rolled with prosciutto or ham (non-nitrate) and a slice of cantaloupe
- Half an apple and 1 tbsp of nut butter (almond, cashew, or macadamia)
- 10 gluten-free crackers (such as Mary's Gone Crackers) with 1 tbsp nut butter
- Gluten-free crackers with snack-sized container of cottage cheese and bunch of black or red grapes, or other fruit
- ¼ cup hummus (organic to avoid GMO oils) with veggies (of mixed colors, such as red peppers, carrots, and snap peas)
- Small square of dark, organic chocolate dipped in natural nut butter
- Fresh salsa with organic black tortilla chips or other multigrain tortilla chips (look for added flax and a fiber content of at least 3 grams)
- ½ avocado with sea salt and drizzle of olive oil and/or balsamic vinegar
- Edamame (make sure to buy non-GMO soybeans)

Road Map to Health: 7 Steps to Alter Your Destination

RESOURCES

I recommend these books, websites, and smartphone apps to help you on your journey to health. Many of the listed authors have multiple books that are worth reading. These are just some of my favorites.

Recommended Reading

Blood Sugar Solution by Mark Hyman, MD

Food Rules by Michael Pollan

Goddesses Never Age by Christiane Northrup, MD

Grain Brain by David Perlmutter, MD

Happy Gut by Vincent Pedre, MD

Immune System Recovery Plan by Susan Blum, MD

New Health Rules by Frank Lipman, MD

Ten Years Younger by Steven Masley, MD

The Disease Delusion by Dr. Jeffrey Bland

The Food Babe Way by Vani Hari

The Sugar Impact Diet by J.J. Virgin

The Wahl's Protocol by Terry Wahls, MD

Wheat Belly by William Davis, MD

Movies

Fat, Sick and Nearly Dead

Food, Inc.

Food Matters

Forks Over Knives

Hungry for Change

Ingredients

Fresh

Supersize Me

Organizations/Websites

Institute for Functional Medicine—Find an FM practitioner
www.functionalmedicine.org

Environmental Defense Fund—Seafood Selector www.seafood.edf.org

Environmental Working Group—Guides for pesticides, cleaning
products, cosmetics, sunscreen www.ewg.org/consumer-guides

Choosing the Right Cooking Oils
www.pccnaturalmarkets.com/guides/tips_cooking_oils.html

Klean Kanteen—nontoxic containers www.kleankanteen.com

Thrive Market—Clean products at wholesale prices
www.thrivemarket.com

Smartphone Apps

Dirty Dozen—Pesticides in produce

Seafood Watch—Clean seafood

Skin Deep—Safer cosmetics

Headspace – Meditation

The 7 Minute Workout – Exercise

ABOUT THE AUTHOR

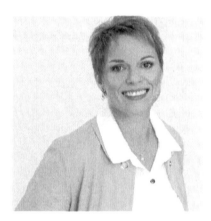

Dr. Robinson was born and raised in Red Bluff, a rural town in northern California. When she entered undergrad at California State University at Long Beach, she only knew that she had a deeply ingrained need to care for people. After she realized that medicine was her calling, she attended Tulane University School of Medicine on an Air Force scholarship, graduating at the top of her class in 1996.

She completed residency at Travis Air Force Base. Being a part of the Air Force was one of the best experiences of her life. She proudly served in the force 1996-2003 and was, caring for our troops, their families, and retired service members.

After her service, she worked in various practice types, all with pressure to attain quantity over quality. Over those years, she came to the sad realization of the futile way in which she was practicing medicine – not enough time with patients leading to more medications and less true healing.

Stacey J. Robinson, MD

In 2008, she opened Robinson MD so she could care for patients in a more thorough, individualized way. Her mission is to empower and inspire patients to achieve their best health. Dr. Robinson is board-certified in Family Medicine and Integrative Medicine. She is also certified in Functional Medicine and a member of the American Academy of Private Physicians.

In her spare time, she enjoys spending time with her family, traveling, spending time outdoors, cooking delicious and nutritious food, photography, and creating beautiful scrapbooks for her family. She lives in St. Petersburg, Florida.

To contact Dr. Robinson or find out more about her practice, visit her website at www.robinsonmed.com.

ENDNOTES

[1] Davis, K., Stremikis, K., Schoen, C., & Squires, D. Mirror, Mirror on the Wall, 2014 Update: How the U.S. Health Care System Compares Internationally. *The Commonwealth Fund*, Jun 2014.

[2] The Henry Kaiser Foundation. Total Number of Retail Prescription Drugs Filled at Pharmacies. Retrieved from http://kff.org/other/state-indicator/total-retail-rx-drugs/

[3] Mayo Clinic News Network. Nearly 7 in 10 Americans Take Prescription Drugs, Mayo Clinic, Olmsted Medical Center Find. Retrevied from http://newsnetwork.mayoclinic.org/discussion/nearly-7-in-10-americans-take-prescription-drugs-mayo-clinic-olmsted-medical-center-find

[4] World Health Organization. Chronic Disease and Health Promotion. Retrieved from http://www.who.int/chp/chronic_disease_report/part1/en/index11.html

[5] Avena, N.M., Rada, P., Bartley, G., & Hoebel, B.G. Evidence for sugar addiction: Behavioral and neurochemical effects of intermittent, excessive sugar intake. *Neuroscience and Biobehavioral Reviews*, 2008; 32(1):20–39.

[6] Hyman, Mark. (2014). Are You Also Being Deceived into Eating Fake Frankenfoods? Retrieved from http://drhyman.com/blog/2010/07/04/are-you-also-being-deceived-into-eating-fake-frankenfoods/

[7] Altschuler, J, Margolius, D, Bodenheimer, T, Grumbach, K. Estimating a Reasonable Patient Panel Size for Primary Care Physicians With Team-Based Task Delegation. *Annals of Family Medicine*, 2012;10(5):396-400.

[8] Rappapport, S,M., Smith, M.T. Environment and disease risks. *Science*, Oct 22 2010; 330: 460-1. doi: 10.1126/science.1192603

[9] Bredeson, D. (2016 Mar 15). 21st Century Medicine and the Reversal of Cognitive Decline in Alzheimer Disease. Cleveland Clinic Grand Rounds, Cleveland, OH.

[10] Bredesen, Dale E., & Easton, Mary S. Center for Alzheimer's Disease Research, Department of Neurology, University of California, Los Angeles, CA. Reversal of cognitive decline: A novel therapeutic program. *Aging*, Sept 2014; Vol 6, No 9:707–717.

[11] Helander, HF, Fändriks, L. Surface area of the digestive tract - revisited. *Scandinavian Journal of Gastroenterology*, Jun 2014; 49(6):681-9. doi: 10.3109/00365521.2014.898326. Epub 2014 Apr 2.

[12] Vighi, G. Marcucci, F., Sensi, L., Di Cara, G., & Frati, F. Allergy and the gastrointestinal system. *Clinical and Experimental Immunology*, 2008 Sep; 153 (Suppl 1): 3–6.

[13] Gershon, M. (1998). *The Second Brain: A Groundbreaking New Understanding of Nervous Disorders of the Stomach and Intestine*. New York, NY. Harper Collins.

[14] Forsythe, P., Bienenstock, J., & Kunze, W.A. Vagal pathways for microbiome-brain-gut axis communication. *Advances in Experimental Medicine and Biology*, 2014; 817:115–133.

[15] Neltner TG, Alger HM, Leonard JE, Maffini MV. Data gaps in toxicity testing of chemicals allowed in food in the United States. *Reproductive Toxicology*, Dec 2013;42:85-94.

[16] Lerner, A. Matthias, T. Changes in intestinal tight junction permeability associated with industrial food additives explain the rising incidence of autoimmune disease. *Autoimmunity Reviews*, Jun 2015, 14:6, 479-489.

[17] Chassaing B, Koren O, Goodrich JK, Poole AC, Srinivasan S, Ley RE, Gewirtz AT. Dietary emulsifiers impact the mouse gut microbiota promoting colitis and metabolic syndrome. Nature. 2015 Mar 5;519 (7541):92-6.

[18] King DE, Mainous AG 3rd, Lambourne CA. Trends in dietary fiber intake in the United States, 1999-2008. *Journal of Academy of Nutrition and Dietetics*. May 2012;112(5):642-8.

[19] Choung RS, Locke GR 3rd, Schleck CD, Zinsmeister AR, Talley NJ. Cumulative incidence of chronic constipation: a population-based study 1988-2003. *Alimentary Pharmacology & Therapeutics*, Dec 2007;26(11-12):1521-8.

[20] Rozing, J., Sapone, A., Lammers, K., & Fasano, A. Tight Junctions, Intestinal Permeability, and Autoimmunity Celiac Disease and Type 1 Diabetes Paradigms. *Annals of the New York Academy of Sciences*, May 2009; 1165:195–205.

[21] Lerner, A., & Matthias, T. Changes in intestinal tight junction permeability associated with industrial food additives explain the rising incidence of autoimmune disease. *Autoimmune Review*, Jun 2015; 14(6):479–489.

[22] Landrigan, P., & Benbrook, C. GMOs, Herbicides, and Public Health. *New England Journal of Medicine*, 2015; 373:693–695.

[23] Herzig SJ, Howell MD, Ngo LH, Marcantonio ER. Acid-suppressive medication use and the risk for hospital-acquired pneumonia. *JAMA*. May 2009; 27;301(20):2120-8. doi: 10.1001/jama.2009.722.

[24] Morrison RH., et al. Risk factors associated with complications and mortality in patients with Clostridium difficile infection. *Clinical Infectious Diseases*. Dec 2011; 53(12):1173-8. doi: 10.1093/cid/cir668. Epub 2011 Oct 5.

[25] Tursi A, Elisei W, Giorgetti GM, Gaspardone A, Lecca PG, Di Cesare L, Brandimarte G. Prevalence of celiac disease and symptoms in relatives of patients with celiac disease.,*European Review for Medical and Pharmacological Sciences*. Jun 2010;14(6):567-72.

[26] The Quotations Page. Accessed at http://www.quotationspage.com/quote/1480.html

[27] Xie, et al. Sleep initiated fluid flux drives metabolite clearance from the adult brain. *Science*, 18 Oct 2013.

[28] Klerk, M., et al. MTHFR 677C→T Polymorphism and Risk of Coronary Heart Disease: A Meta-analysis. *JAMA*, 2002; 288(16):2023-2031. doi:10.1001/jama.288.16.2023.

[29] Gilbody, S., Lewis, S., Lightfoot, T. Methylenetetrahydrofolate Reductase (MTHFR) Genetic Polymorphisms and Psychiatric Disorders: A HuGE Review. *American Journal of Epidemiology*, 2007; 165(1): 1-13.

[30] Wu, Y.L., Ding X.X., Sun Y.H., Sun L. Methylenetetrahydrofolate reductase (MTHFR) C677T/A1298C polymorphisms and susceptibility to Parkinson's disease: A meta-analysis. *Journal of Neurological Sciences*, 2013; 335(1-2):14-21. doi: 10.1016/j.jns.2013.09.006. Epub 2013 Sep 12.

[31] Blaha, M.J., Budoff, M.J., DeFilippis, A.P., et al. Associations between C-reactive protein, coronary artery calcium, and cardiovascular events: implications for the JUPITER population from MESA, a population-based cohort study. *Lancet,* 2011; 378:684–692.

[32] Oyebode, O., Gordon-Dseagu, B., Walker, A., & Mindell, J.S. Fruit and vegetable consumption and all-cause cancer and CVD mortality: analysis of Health Survey for England data. *Journal of Epidemiology and Community Health*, 31 Mar 2014; doi:10.1136/jech-2013-203500.

[33] National Institutes of Health. Estimates of Funding for Various Research, Condition, and Disease Categories (RCDC). (February 10, 2016). Retrieved from https://report.nih.gov/categorical_spending.aspx.

[34] CNN Wire Staff. (Oct 26, 2010). Everyday Chemicals May Be Harming Kids, Panel Told. Retrieved from http://www.cnn.com/2010/HEALTH/10/26/senate.toxic.america.hearing/.

[35] Neltner, T., Alger, H., Leonard, J. Maffini, M. Data gaps in toxicity testing of chemicals allowed in food in the United States. *Reproductive Toxicology*. Dec 2013; Volume 42; Pages 85–94.

[36] Zhiwei Hu, et al. Assessing the carcinogenic potential of low-dose exposures to chemical mixtures in the environment: the challenge ahead. *Carcinogenesis*, 2015; 36 (Suppl 1).

[37] Spalding, KL., Bhardwaj, RD, Buchholz, BA, Frisen, J. Retrospective birth dating of cells in humans. Cell. Jul 15 2005;122(1):133-43.

[38] Pollan, M. (2009) Food Rules: An Eater's Manuel. New York, NY: Penguin Books.

[39] Pollan, M. (2009). In Defense of Food: An Eater's Manifesto. New York, NY: Penguin Books.

[40] U.S. Food & Drug Administration. (2015). AquAdvantage Salmon. Retrieved from http://www.fda.gov/AnimalVeterinary/DevelopmentApprovalProcess/GeneticEngineering/GeneticallyEngineeredAnimals/ucm280853.htm

[41] Landrigan, P., & Benbrook, C. Gmos, Herbicides, and Public Health. *New England Journal of Medicine*, 2015; 373:693–695.

[42] Jotham Suez, et al. Artificial sweeteners induce glucose intolerance by altering the gut microbiota. *Nature*, 09 Oct 2014; 514:181–186.

[43] Mcbride, Judy. (Nov 20, 1996). USDA Finds More and More Americans Eat Out, Offers Tips for Making Healthier Food Choices. Retrieved from http://www.ars.usda.gov/is/pr/1996/eatout1196.htm

[44] Fruit and vegetable consumption and mortality from all causes, cardiovascular disease, and cancer: systematic review and dose-response meta-analysis of prospective cohort studies. *BMJ*, 2014; 349:g4490.

[45] Esselstyn Jr, C.B., Gendy, G., Doyle, J., Golubic, M., & Roizen, M.F. A Way to Reverse CAD. *The Journal of Family Practice*, Jul 2014; Vol 63, No 7.

[46] Memorial Sloan Kettering Cancer Center, Integrative Medicine, Herbs and Botanicals. Accessed on 07 Sept 2015. https://www.mskcc.org/cancer-care/treatments/symptom-management/integrative-medicine/herbs/search.

[47] Fleischauer, A.T., Poole, C., & Arab, L. Garlic consumption and cancer prevention: meta-analyses of colorectal and stomach cancers. *The American Journal of Clinical Nutrition*, Oct 2000; 72(4):1047–1052.

[48] Laidlaw, M., Cockerline, C.A., & Sepkovic, D.W. Effects of a breast-health herbal formula supplement on estrogen metabolism in pre- and post-

menopausal women not taking hormonal contraceptives or supplements: a randomized controlled trial. *Breast Cancer*, 16 Dec 2010; 4:85–95.

[49] Nachshon-Kedmi, M., et al. Indole-3-carbinol and 3,3'-diindolylmethane induce apoptosis in human prostate cancer cells. *Food and Chemical Toxicology*, Jun 2003; 41(6):745–752.

[50] Royston, K.J., & Tollefsbol, T.O. The Epigenetic Impact of Cruciferous Vegetables on Cancer Prevention. *Current Pharmacology Reports.*, 01 Feb 2015; 1(1):46–51.

[51] Abdulah, R., Faried, A., Kobayashi, K., et al. Selenium enrichment of broccoli sprout extract increases chemosensitivity and apoptosis of LNCaP prostate cancer cells. *BMC Cancer*, 2009; 9:414.

[52] Li, Y., Zhang, T., Korkaya, H., et al. Sulforaphane, a dietary component of broccoli/broccoli sprouts, inhibits breast cancer stem cells. *Clinical Cancer Research*, 2010; 16(9):2580–2590.

[53] Hsu, S.D., et al. Chemoprevention of oral cancer by green tea. *General Dentistry*, 2002; 50:140–146.

[54] Pisters, K.M., et al. Phase I trial of oral green tea extract in adult patients with solid tumors. *Journal of Clinical Oncology*, 2001; 19:1830–1838.

[55] Proniuk, S., et al. Preformulation study of epigallocatechin gallate, a promising antioxidant for topical skin cancer prevention. *Journal of Pharmaceutical Sciences*, 2002; 91:111–116.

[56] Sartippour, M.R., et al. Green tea inhibits vascular endothelial growth factor (VEGF) induction in human breast cancer cells. *Journal of Nutrition*, 2002; 132:2307–2311.

[57] Sun, C.L., et al. Urinary tea polyphenols in relation to gastric and esophageal cancers: a prospective study of men in Shanghai, China. *Carcinogenesis*, 2002; 23:1497–1503.

58 Nechuta, S., Shu, X.O., Li, H.L., et al. Prospective cohort study of tea consumption and risk of digestive system cancers: results from the Shanghai Women's Health Study. *American Journal of Clinical Nutrition*, Nov 2012; 96(5):1056–1063. doi:10.3945/ajcn.111.031419. Epub 10 Oct 2012.

59 Anti, M., Armelao, F., Marra, G., Percesepe, A., Bartoli, G.M., Palozza, P., et al. Effects of different doses of fish oil on rectal cell proliferation in patients with sporadic colonic adenomas. *Gastroenterology,* 1994; 107:1709–18.

60 Wolk, A., Larsson, S.C., Johansson, J., & Ekman, P. Long-term fatty fish consumption and renal cell carcinoma incidence in women. *Journal of the American Medical Association*, 2006; 296(11):1371–1376.

61 Brasky, T.M., Lampe, J.W., Potter, J.D., Patterson, R.E., & White, E. Specialty Supplements and Breast Cancer Risk in the VITamins and Lifestyle (VITAL) Cohort. *Cancer Epidemiology, Biomarkers & Prevention*, 2010; 19(7):1696–1708.

62 U.S. Food and Drug Administration. (July 1999). Health Claim Notification for Whole Grain Foods. Retrieved from http://www.fda.gov/Food/IngredientsPackagingLabeling/LabelingNutrition/ucm073639.htm

63 Halyburton, A.K., et al. Low- and high-carbohydrate weight-loss diets have similar effects on mood but not cognitive performance. *American Journal of Clinical Nutrition*, Sep 2007:86(3); 580-7.

64 Keogh, J.B., et al. Effects of weight loss from a very-low-carbohydrate diet on endothelial function and markers of cardiovascular disease risk in subjects with abdominal obesity. *American Journal of Clinical Nutrition*, Mar 2008; 87(3); 567-76.

65 Brinkworth, G.D., et al. Long-term effects of a very-low-carbohydrate weight loss diet compared with an isocaloric low-fat diet after 12 months. *American Journal of Clinical Nutrition*, Jul 2009: 90(1); 23-32.

Stacey J. Robinson, MD

[66] Hernandez, T.L. et al. Lack of suppression of circulating free fatty acids and hypercholesterolemia during weight loss on a high-fat, low-carbohydrate diet. *American Journal of Clinical Nutrition*, Mar 2010: 91(3); 578-85.

[67] Foster, G.D., et al. A Randomized Trial of a Low-Carbohydrate Diet for Obesity. *New England Journal of Medicine,* 2003; 348:2082–2090.

[68] Samaha, F.F., et al. A Low-Carbohydrate as Compared with a Low-Fat Diet in Severe Obesity. *New England Journal of Medicine,* 2003; 348:2074–2081.

[69] Shai, I., et al. Weight loss with a low-carbohydrate, Mediterranean, or low-fat diet. *New England Journal of Medicine*, Jul 2008: 359; 229-41.

[70] Brehm, B.J., Seeley, R.J., Daniels, S.R., & D'Alessio, D.A. A Randomized Trial Comparing a Very Low Carbohydrate Diet and a Calorie-Restricted Low Fat Diet on Body Weight and Cardiovascular Risk Factors in Healthy Women. *The Journal of Clinical Endocrinology & Metabolism*, Jan 2003; 88(4):1617–1623.

[71] Meckling, K.A., O'Sullivan, C., Saari, D. Comparison of a low-fat diet to a low-carbohydrate diet on weight loss, body composition, and risk factors for diabetes and cardiovascular disease in free-living, overweight men and women. *The Journal of Clinical Endocrinology & Metabolism*, Jun 2004: 89(6); 2717-23.

[72] Daly, M.E., et al. Short-term effects of severe dietary carbohydrate-restriction advice in Type 2 diabetes. *Diabetic Medicine*, Jan 2006: 23(1): 15-20.

[73] Dyson, P.A., et al. A low-carbohydrate diet is more effective in reducing body weight than healthy eating in both diabetic and non-diabetic subjects. *Diabetic Medicine*, 2007.

[74] Krebs, N.F., et al. Efficacy and safety of a high protein, low carbohydrate diet for weight loss in severely obese adolescents. *Journal of Pediatrics*, Aug 2010: 157(2); 252-8.

[75] Sondike, S.B., Copperman, N., & Jacobson, M.S. Effects of a low-carbohydrate diet on weight loss and cardiovascular risk factor in overweight adolescents. *The Journal of Pediatrics*, Mar 2003; Vol 142, Issue 3:253–258.

[76] Volek, J.S., et al. Comparison of energy-restricted very low-carbohydrate and low-fat diets on weight loss and body composition in overweight men and women. *Nutrition & Metabolism* (London), Nov 2004: 1(1); 13.

[77] Westman, E.C., Yancy Jr., W.S., Mavropoulos, J.C., Marquart, M., McDuffie, J.R. The effect of a low-carbohydrate, ketogenic diet versus a low-glycemic index diet on glycemic control in type 2 diabetes mellitus. *Nutrition & Metabolism* (London), Dec 2008: 5;36.

[78] Aude, Y.W., Agatston, A.S., Lopez-Jimenez, F., Lieberman, E.H., Marie Almon, Hansen, M., Rojas, G., Lamas, G.A., & Hennekens, C.H. The national cholesterol education program diet vs a diet lower in carbohydrates and higher in protein and monounsaturated fat: a randomized trial. *Archives of Internal Medicine*, 25 Oct 2004; 164(19):2141–2146.

[79] Yancy Jr., W.S., Olsen, M.K., Guyton, J.R., Bakst, R.P., Westman, E.C. A low-carbohydrate, ketogenic diet versus a low-fat diet to treat obesity and hyperlipidemia. *Annals of Internal Medicine*, May 2004: 140(10); 769-72.

[80] Nickols-Richardson, S.M., et al. Perceived hunger is lower and weight loss is greater in overweight premenopausal women consuming a low-carbohydrate/high-protein vs high-carbohydrate/low-fat diet. *Journal of the American Dietetic Association*, Sep 2005: 105(9); 1433-7.

[81] Mcclernon, F.J., et al. The effects of a low-carbohydrate ketogenic diet and a low-fat diet on mood, hunger, and other self-reported symptoms. *Obesity* (Silver Spring), Jan 2007: 15(1); 182-7.

[82] Gardner, C.D., et al. Comparison of the Atkins, Zone, Ornish, and LEARN diets for change in weight and related risk factors among overweight premenopausal women: the A TO Z Weight Loss Study. *Journal of the American Medical Association*, Mar 2007: 297(9); 969-77.

[83] Tay, J., Brinkworth, G.D., Noakes, M., Keogh, J., Clifton, P.M. Metabolic effects of weight loss on a very-low-carbohydrate diet compared with an isocaloric high-carbohydrate diet in abdominally obese subjects. *Journal of the American College of Cardiology*, Jan 2008: 51(1); 59-67.

Stacey J. Robinson, MD

84 Volek, J.S., et al. Carbohydrate restriction has a more favorable impact on the metabolic syndrome than a low fat diet. *Lipids*, Apr 2009: 44(4); 297-309.

85 Guldbrand H., et al. In type 2 diabetes, randomization to advice to follow a low-carbohydrate diet transiently improves glycaemic control compared with advice to follow a low-fat diet producing a similar weight loss. *Diabetologia*, Aug 2012: 55(8); 2118-27.

86 Willett, W.C. Dietary fat intake and cancer risk: a controversial and instructive story. *Seminars in Cancer Biology*, Aug 1998; 8(4):245–253.

87 Salas-Salvado, J., et al. Reduction in the incidence of type 2 diabetes with the Mediterranean diet: results of the PREDIMED-Reusnutrition intervention randomized trial. *Diabetes Care*, 2011; 34(1): 14-9.

88 Toledo, E., et al. Mediterranean Diet and Invasive Breast Cancer Risk Among Women at High Cardiovascular Risk in the PREDIMED Trial: A Randomized Clinical Trial. *JAMA Internal Medicine*, 2015; 175 (11): 1752-60.

89 Fernandez-Castillejo, S., et al. Polyphenol rich olive oils improve lipoprotein particle atherogenic ratios and subclasses profile: a randomized, crossover, controlled trial. *Molecular Nutrition & Food Research*, 2016; doi: 10.1002/mnfr.201501068. [Epub ahead of print]

90 Medina-Remon, A., et al. Polyphenol intake from a Mediterranean diet decreases inflammatory biomarkers related to atherosclerosis: A sub-study of The PREDIMED trial. *British Journal of Clinical Pharmacology*, 2016; doi: 10.1111/bcp.12986. [Epub ahead of print]

91 Martinez-Gonzalez, M.A., et al. Benefits of the Mediterranean Diet: Insights From the PREDIMED Study. *Progress in Cardiovascular Disease*, 2015; 58(1); 50-60.

92 Moral, R., Escrich, R., Solanas, M., Vela, E., Ruiz de Villa, M.C., & Escrich, E. Diets high in corn oil or extra-virgin olive oil differentially modify the gene expression profile of the mammary gland and influence experimental breast cancer susceptibility. *European Journal of Nutrition*, Jun 2016: 55(4); 1397-409. doi: 10.1007/s00394-015-0958-2. Epub 2015 Jun 20.

[93] Perlmutter, D. (Sep 14, 2012). Mitochondrial Therapeutics in Neurodegenerative Disease. Applying Functional Medicine in Clinical Practice, Institute for Functional Medicine.

[94] Research shows eggs from pastured chickens may be more nutritious. Penn State News. Penn State's Dairy Cattle Research and Education Center, 20 July 2010. http://news.psu.edu/story/166143/2010/07/20/research-shows-eggs-pastured-chickens-may-be-more-nutritious.

[95] Goodrow, E.F., et al. Consumption of one egg per day increases serum lutein and zeaxanthin concentrations in older adults without altering serum lipid and lipoprotein cholesterol concentrations. *Journal of Nutrition*, Oct 2006; 136(10):2519–2524.

[96] Wenzel, A.J., Gerweck, C., Barbato, D., Nicolosi, R.J., Handelman, G.J., & Curran-Celentano, J.A. 12-wk egg intervention increases serum zeaxanthin and macular pigment optical density in women. *Journal of Nutrition*, Oct 2006; 136(10):2568–2573.

[97] Blesso, C.N., Andersen, C.J., Barona, J., Volek, J., & Fernandez, M.L. Whole egg consumption improves lipoprotein profiles and insulin sensitivity in individuals with metabolic syndrome. *Metabolism,* 2013; 62:400–410.

[98] Ying Rong, et al. Egg consumption and risk of coronary heart disease and stroke: dose-response meta-analysis of prospective cohort studies. *BMJ,* 2013; 346:e8539

[99] Perlmutter, David. Your Brain Needs Cholesterol. Retrieved from http://www.drperlmutter.com/brain-needs-cholesterol/

[100] Scientific Report of the 2015 Dietary Guidelines Advisory Committee. (2015). Cholesterol not a nutrient of concern. Retrieved from http://health.gov/dietaryguidelines/2015-scientific-report/.

[101] Greenland, P., LaBree, L., Azen, S.P., Doherty, T.M., & Detrano, R.C. Coronary Artery Calcium Score Combined With Framingham Score for Risk Prediction in

Asymptomatic Individuals. *Journal of the American Medical Association*, 2004; 291(2):210–215.

[102] Polonsky, T.S., et al. Coronary Artery Calcium Score and Risk Classification for Coronary Heart Disease Prediction. *Journal of the American Medical Association*, 2010; 303(16):1610–1616. doi:10.1001/jama.2010.461.

[103] Shaw, L.J., Raggi, P., Schisterman, E., Berman, D.S., & Callister, T.Q. Prognostic Value of Cardiac Risk Factors and Coronary Artery Calcium Screening for All-Cause Mortality. *Radiology*, 2003; 228(3):826–833.

[104] Taylor, A.J., et al. Coronary Calcium Independently Predicts Incident Premature Coronary Heart Disease Over Measured Cardiovascular Risk Factors. *Journal of the American College of Cardiology,* 2005; 46(5):807–814. doi:10.1016/j.jacc.2005.05.049.

[105] Church, T., et al. Coronary artery calcium score, risk factors, and incident coronary heart disease events. *Atherosclerosis*, 2007; 190(1):224–231.

[106] Zero coronary calcium means very low 10-year event risk. *Family Practice News*, 16 Jan 2015. http://www.familypracticenews.com/home/article/zero-coronary-calcium-means-very-low-10-year-event-risk/b45e3dadd4a19ca1907d20dcccd877e5.html?ooct=FPN-related.

[107] Buitrago, F. et al. Original and REGICOR Framingham Functions in a Nondiabetic Population of a Spanish Health Care Center: A Validation Study. *Annals of Family Medicine.* 2011 Sep; 9(5): 431–438.

[108] Sung, J. et al. Diagnostic Value of Coronary Artery Calcium Score for Cardiovascular Disease in African Americans: The Jackson Heart Study. *British Journal of Medicine and Medical Research.* 2016,;11(2). pii: BJMMR/2016/21449. Epub 2015 Sep 21.

[109] Cederberg, H., Stančáková, A., Yaluri, N., Modi, S., Kuusisto, J., & Laakso, M. Increased risk of diabetes with statin treatment is associated with impaired insulin sensitivity and insulin secretion: a 6-year follow-up study of the METSIM cohort. *Diabetologia*, May 2015; 58(5):1109–1117.

[110] Davis, D.R., Epp, M.D., Riordan, H.D. Changes in USDA food composition data for 43 garden crops, 1950 to 1999. *Journal of the American College of Nutrition*, Dec 2004;23(6):669-82.

[111] Uedo, N. et al. Reduction in salivary cortisol level by music therapy during colonoscopic examination. *Hepatogastroenterology.* 2004 Mar-Apr;51(56): 451-453.

[112] Samel, A., Vejvoda, M., Maass, H. Sleep deficit and stress hormones in helicopter pilots on 7-day duty for emergency medical services. *Aviation, Space and Environmental Medicine*, Nov 2004;75(11): 935-40.

[113] Bains, G.S, Berk, L.S, Daher, N., Lohman, E., Schwab, E., Petrofsky, J., Deshpande, P., The effect of humor on short-term memory in older adults: a new component for whole-person wellness. *Advances in Mind-Body Medicine*; Spring 2014; 28(2): 16-24.

[114] Field, T., Hernandez-Reif, M., Diego, M., Schanberg, S., Kuhn, C. Cortisol decreases and serotonin and dopamine increase following massage therapy. *International Journal of Neuroscience*, Oct 2005, 115(10), 1397-413.

[115] Lovallo, W.R, Whitsett, T.L., al Absi, M., Sung, B.H., Vincent, A.S., Wilson, M.F. Caffeine Stimulation of Cortisol Secretion Across the Waking Hours in Relation to Caffeine Intake Levels. *Psychosomatic Medicine*, 2005; 67(5): 734-739.

[116] Maclean, CR et al. Effects of the Transcendental Meditation program on adaptive mechanisms: changes in hormone levels and responses to stress after 4 months of practice. *Psychoneuroendocrinology*. 1997 May;22(4): 277-95.

[117] Hansen, J., & Lassen, C.F. Nested case-control study of night shift work and breast cancer risk among women in the Danish military. *Occupational and Environmental Medicine*, Aug 2012; 69(8):551–556.

[118] Sigurdardottir, Lara, et al. Sleep Disruption Among Older Men and Risk of Prostate Cancer. *Cancer Epidemiology, Biomarkers & Prevention*, 22 May 2013; 872.

[119] Thompson, Larkin E.K., Patel, S., Berger, N.A., Redline, S., & Li, L. Short duration of sleep increases risk of colorectal adenoma. *Cancer*, 15 Feb 2011; 117(4):841–847.

[120] Sephton, S. Circadian Disruption in Cancer: a neuroendocrine pathway from stress to disease. *Brain, Behavior and Immunity*, Oct 2003; Vol. 17:321–328.

[121] Hakim, F., et al. Fragmented sleep accelerates tumor growth and progression through recruitment of tumor-associated macrophages and TLR4 signaling. *Cancer Research*, 01 Mar 2014; 74(5):1329–1337.

[122] Cappuccio, F.P., Cooper, D., D'Elia, L., Strazzullo, P., & Miller, M.A. Sleep duration predicts cardiovascular outcomes: a systematic review and meta-analysis of prospective studies. *The European Heart Journal*, Jun 2011; 32(12):1484–1492.

[123] Hublin, C., Partinen, M., Koskenvuo, M., & Kaprio, J. Sleep and mortality: a population-based 22-year follow-up study. *Sleep*, 01 Oct 2007; 30(10):1245–1571.

[124] Barefoot, John, et al. Recovery Expectations and Long-term Prognosis of Patients with Coronary Heart Disease. *Archives of Internal Medicine*, 2011; 171(10):929–935.

[125] Yanek, Lisa R. Effect of Positive Well-Being on Incidence of Symptomatic Coronary Artery Disease. *American Journal of Cardiology*, 15 October 2013; Vol 112, Issue 8:1120–1125.

[126] Ostir, G.V., Ottenbacher, K.J., Markides, K.C.. Onset of frailty in older adults and the protective role of positive affect. . *Psychology and Aging*, Sep 2004; 29(3); 402-8.

[127] Levy, B.R., Slade, M.D., Kunkel, S.R., & Kasl, S.V. Longevity increased by positive self-perceptions of aging. *Journal of Personality and Social Psychology*, Aug 2002; 83(2):261–270.

[128] Koyama, Tetsuo, McHaffie, John G., Laurienti, Paul J., & Coghill, Robert C. The subjective experience of pain: Where expectations become reality. *Proceedings of the National Academy of Sciences of the United States of America*, 2005; 102(36)12950–12955.

[129] Berger, M.M., et al. Impact of a pain protocol including hypnosis in major burns. *Burns*, Aug 2010; 36(5):639–646.

[130] Spiegel, D. The Mind Prepared: Hypnosis in Surgery. *Journal of the National Cancer Institute*, 2007; 99(17):1280–1281.

[131] Williams, J.E., Paton, C.C., Siegler, I.C., Eigenbrodt, M.L., Nieto, F.J., & Tyroler, H.A. Anger proneness predicts coronary heart disease risk: prospective analysis from the atherosclerosis risk in communities (ARIC) study. *Circulation*, 02 May 2000; 101(17):2034–2039.

[132] Brainy Quote. Retrieved from http://www.brainyquote.com/quotes/quotes/m/mahatmagan121411.html.

[133] Pillemer, K., Fuller-Rowell, T.E., Reid, M.C., & Wells, N.M. Environmental Volunteering and Health Outcomes over a 20-Year Period. *Gerontologist*, Oct 2010; 50(5):594–602.

[134] Patel, A.V., et al. Leisure time spent sitting in relation to total mortality in a prospective cohort of US adults. *American Journal of Epidemiology*, 15 Aug 2010; 172(4):419–429.

[135] Warburton, D.E., Whitney, Nicol C., & Bredin, S. Health benefits of physical activity: the evidence. *Canadian Medical Association Journal*, 2006; 174(6):801–809.

[136] Arem, H., et al. Leisure time physical activity and mortality: a detailed pooled analysis of the dose-response relationship. *JAMA Internal Medicine*, Jun 2015; 175(6):959–967.

[137] Norton, S., Matthews, F.E., Barnes, D.E., Yaffe, K., & Brayne, C. Potential for primary prevention of Alzheimer's disease: an analysis of population-based data. *The Lancet Neurology*, Aug 2014; 13(8):788–794.

[138] Goldsmith, S., et al. Improving Quality of Life of Older Adults Through a Hospital-based Exercise Program. Public & Patient Education Department, Education & Academic Affairs, Hospital for Special Surgery, New York, New York, 15 Dec 2014. https://www.hss.edu/newsroom_hospital-based-exercise-program-improves-quality-of-life-adult-arthritis.asp.

[139] Craft, L.L., & Perna, F.M. The Benefits of Exercise for the Clinically Depressed. Prim Care Companion. *Journal of Clinical Psychiatry*, 2004; 6(3):104–111.

[140] Center for Disease Control and Prevention. (2015). National Center for Health Statistics. Retrieved from http://www.cdc.gov/nchs/fastats/exercise.htm.

[141] Hambrecht, R., et al. Percutaneous Coronary Angioplasty Compared With Exercise Training in Patients with Stable Coronary Artery Disease. *Circulation*, 2004; 109(11):1371–1378.

[142] Pandey, A. et al. Dose-Response Relationship Between Physical Activity and Risk of Heart Failure: A Meta-Analysis. *Circulation*, Nov 10 2015; 132(19): 1786-94.

[143] Talanian, J., Galloway, S.D., Heigenhauser, G.J., Bonen, A., & Spriet, L.L. Two weeks of high-intensity aerobic interval training increases the capacity for fat oxidation during exercise in women. *Journal of Applied Physiology*, 01 April 2007; Vol 102, No. 4:1439–1447.

[144] Heydari, M., Freund, J., & Boutcher, S.H. The effect of high-intensity intermittent exercise on body composition of overweight young males. *Journal of Obesity*, 2012; Article ID 480467.

145 Airin, S. The Effects of High-Intensity Interval Training and Continuous Training on Weight Loss and Body Composition in Overweight Females. *Proceedings of the International Colloquium on Sports Science, Exercise, Engineering and Technology,* 29 Jul 2014; 401–409.

146 Stokes, K.A., Nevill, M.E., Hall, G.M., Lakomy, H.K. The time course of the human growth hormone response to a 6 s and a 30 s cycle ergometer sprint. *Journal of Sports Science,* 2002; 32(15): 987-1004.

147 Shaban, N., Kenno, K.A., Milne, K.J. The effects of a 2 week modified high intensity interval training program on the homeostatic model of insulin resistance (HOMA-IR) in adults with type 2 diabetes. *Journal of Sports Medicine and Physical Fitness,* Jun 2002; 20(6): 487-94.

148 Robinson, S. Patient records from private practice, 2008-2014 inclusive.

149 Vitamin D and Health, The Nutrition Source, Harvard School of Public Health. Accessed 29 August 2015.
http://www.hsph.harvard.edu/nutritionsource/vitamin-d/.

150 National Academics of Science, Engineering and Medicine. (Nov 30 2010). Dietary Reference Intakes for Calcium and Vitamin D. Retrieved from http://www.nationalacademies.org/hmd/Reports/2010/Dietary-Reference-Intakes-for-Calcium-and-Vitamin-D/Report-Brief.aspx.

151 Painter, Kim. (2013, February 25). Calcium, vitamin D get thumbs-down from task force. Retrieved from http://www.usatoday.com/story/news/nation/2013/02/25/calcium-vitamins-bone-fractures/1946661/.

152 Moyer, V.A. Vitamin D and Calcium Supplementation to Prevent Fractures in Adults: U.S. Preventive Services Task Force Recommendation Statement. *Annals of Internal Medicine,* 2013; 158(9): 691-696.

Stacey J. Robinson, MD

[153] Bischoff-Ferrari, H., et al. Fracture Prevention With Vitamin D Supplementation. A Meta-analysis of Randomized Controlled Trials. *Journal of the American Medical Association*, 2005; 293(18):2257–2264.

[154] Bischoff-Ferrari, H.A. Fall prevention with supplemental and active forms of vitamin D: a meta-analysis of randomised controlled trials. *British Medical Journal*, 2009; 339:b3692.

[155] Bischoff-Ferrari, H.A., Giovannucci, E., Willett, W.C., Dietrich, T., Dawson-Hughes, B. Estimation of optimal serum concentrations of 25-hydroxyvitamin D for multiple health outcomes. *American Journal of Clinical Nutrition*, July 2006;84(1):18-28.

[156] Garland, C.F., Gorham, E.D., Mohr, S.B., Garland, F.C. Vitamin D for cancer prevention: global perspective. *Annals of Epidemiology*, July 2009;19(7):468-83. doi: 10.1016/j.annepidem.2009.03.021.

[157] McDonnell, S.L. et al. Incidence rate of type 2 diabetes is >50% lower in GrassrootsHealth cohort with median serum 25-hydroxyvitamin D of 41 ng/ml than in NHANES cohort with median of 22 ng/ml. *Journal of Steroid Biochemistry and Molecular Biology*, January 2016;155(Pt B):239-44. doi: 10.1016/j.jsbmb.2015.06.013. Epub 2015 Jul 4.

[158] Mohr, S.B., Gorham, E.D., Kim, J., Hoffich, H., Garland, C.F. Meta-analysis of vitamin D sufficiency for improving survival of patients with breast cancer. *Anticancer Research*, March 2014;34(3):1163-6.

[159] Mohr, S.B., Gorham, E.D., Kim, J., Hoffich, H., Cuomo, R.E., Garland, C.F. Could vitamin D sufficiency improve the survival of colorectal cancer patients? *Journal of Steroid Biochemistry and Molecular Biology*, April 2015;148:239-44. doi: 10.1016/j.jsbmb.2014.12.010. Epub 2014 Dec 19.

[160] Tripkovic, L., Lambert, H., Hart, K., et al. Comparison of vitamin D_2 and vitamin D_3 supplementation in raising serum 25-hydroxyvitamin D status: a systematic review and meta-analysis. *American Journal of Clinical Nutrition*, Jun 2012: 95(6); 1357-64. doi: 10.3945/ajcn.111.031070. Epub 2012 May 2.

[161] Logan, V.F., Gray, A.R., Peddie, M.C., et al. Long-term vitamin D_3 supplementation is more effective than vitamin D_2 in maintaining serum 25-

hydroxyvitamin D status over the winter months. *British Journal of Nutrition*, 2013; 109:1082–1088.

[162] Lehmann, U., Hirche, F., Stangl, G.I., et al. Bioavailability of vitamin D(2) and D(3) in healthy volunteers, a randomized placebo-controlled trial. *Journal of Clinical Endocrinology & Metabolism*, 2013; 98:4339–4345.

[163] Holmberg, I., Berlin, T., Ewerth, S., et al. 25-Hydroxylase activity in subcellular fractions from human liver. Evidence for different rates of mitochondrial hydroxylation of vitamin D_2 and D_3. *Scandinavian Journal of Clinical & Laboratory Investigation*, 1986; 46:785–790.

[164] Houghton, L.A., & Vieth, R. The case against ergocalciferol (vitamin D_2) as a vitamin supplement. *American Journal of Clinical Nutrition*, 2006; 84:694–697.

[165] Palmer, Julie R., et al. Onset of Natural Menopause in African American women. *American Journal of Public Health*, Feb 2003; 93(2):299–306.

[166] Nelson, R.J. Hormones & Behavior. The Ohio State University. Retrieved from http://nobaproject.com/modules/hormones-behavior.

[167] Jellinger, P.S. Metabolic consequences of hyperglycemia and insulin resistance. *Clinical Cornerstone*, 2007; 8 Suppl 7:S30–S42.

[168] Hamburg, M.A. (2012, November 15). Pharmacy Compounding: Implications of the 2012 Meningitis Outbreak. Retrieved from http://www.fda.gov/NewsEvents/Testimony/ucm327667.htm.

[169] Writing Group for the Women's Health Initiative Investigators. Risks and Benefits of Estrogen Plus Progestin in Healthy Postmenopausal Women Principal Results From the Women's Health Initiative Randomized Controlled Trial. *JAMA*, 2002; 288(3):321-333.

[170] Holtorf, K. The bioidentical hormone debate: are bioidentical hormones (estradiol, estriol, and progesterone) safer or more efficacious than commonly

used synthetic versions in hormone replacement therapy? *Postgraduate Medicine,* Jan 2009; 121(1):73–85.

[171] Tutera, G. Marked reduction of breast, endometrial and ovarian cancer in users of bio-identical estradiol and testosterone subcutaneous pellets. *Maturitas,* 2009; 63 Suppl 1:S1–S136.

[172] Traish, A.M., Haider, A., Doros, G., & Saad, F. Long-term testosterone therapy in hypogonadal men ameliorates elements of the metabolic syndrome: an observational, long-term registry study. *International Journal of Clinical Practice,* 2013. doi:10.1111/ijcp.12319.

[173] Morgentaler, A. Testosterone Therapy and Cardiovascular Risk: Advances and Controversies. *Mayo Clinic Proceedings,* Feb 2015; 90(20):224–251.

[174] Morgentaler, A. Testosterone and prostate cancer: an historical perspective on a modern myth. *European Urology,* Nov 2006; 50(5):935–939. Epub 27 Jul 2006.

[175] Dupree, J.M., Langille, G.M., Khera, M., & Lipshultz, L.I. The safety of testosterone supplementation therapy in prostate cancer. *Nature Reviews Urology,* Jul 2014; 11:526–530.

Road Map to Health: 7 Steps to Alter Your Destination

Made in the USA
Columbia, SC
18 September 2018